D0815941

Unlocking the Heart Chakra

Unlocking the Heart Chakra

Heal Your Relationships with Love

DR. BRENDA DAVIES

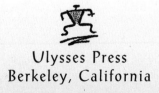

Ulysses Press
Berkeley, California

Published by: Ulysses Press
P.O. Box 3440
Berkeley, CA 94703
www.ulyssespress.com

Library of Congress Catalog Card Number: 00-107043

ISBN: 1-56975-245-1

First published in the United Kingdom as *Affairs of the Heart* in 2000 by Hodder & Stoughton, a division of Hodder Headline PLC

Printed in Canada by Transcontinental Printing

10 9 8 7 6 5 4 3 2 1

Editorial and production staff: Lily Chou, Marin Van Young, David Wells
Book Design: Sarah Levin
Cover Photograph: SuperStock

Distributed in the United States by Publishers Group West

This book has been written and published strictly for informational purposes, and in no way should be used as a substitute for consultation with health care professionals. You should not consider educational material herein to be the practice of medicine or to replace consultation with a physician or other medical practitioner. The author and publisher are providing you with information in this work so that you can have the knowledge and can choose, at your own risk, to act on that knowledge. The author and publisher also urge all readers to be aware of their health status and to consult health professionals before beginning any health program, including changes in dietary habits.

To my mother and father, Hilda and Tom Todd,
who were my first teachers of love.
To my children, Keith and Lesda,
who are living proof of love.
To Elizabeth, my daughter-in-law,
who demonstrates love.
To Jonathan, my grandson,
who embodies love.
To my soul mate whom I shall always love
and all those I have loved in whatever capacity.

ACKNOWLEDGMENTS

*T*here are so many people who have once again helped me bring together my thoughts and help birth this book. Though they are too many to mention, some particularly come to mind, and I send them all my heartfelt thanks.

My lovely mother, who from her nursing home researched poetry and quotations and as always cheered me on my way, assuring me of her love for me—as though I could ever forget. My father, no longer on the earthly plane, but with me every day. My children Lesda and Keith and daughter-in-law Elizabeth for their love and support. Jonathan for walks on the Yorkshire moors and cuddles that made new again the sweet innocence love of childhood. My sister, Pam, with whom I'm still working out things about love; our relationship has taught me much. My wonderful friends Ewa Walker and Del McNeil for their love and their healing, and Scott Hunt, once assistant, now cherished friend, with whom I've been on many a journey before, and who heals me with love and laughter. Nigel Shakespeare, my secretary, who has soothed and supported me throughout with kind words and cups of tea, and Patricia Hodgkinson and the staff of Charter Nightingale Hospital and Edward House in London who have supported my work for many years. My friend Annie Lionnet, who eloquently translated the astrological aspects that at times left me floundering, and reminded me that being plunged into chaos is sometimes the only way to reconstruct cosmos. Claire Gilman, my editor for *Rainbow Journey*, who has become a dear and supportive friend. Ian Robson, who so patiently talked me through a technological crisis over the phone across the Atlantic. Cheryl van Blerk, who supports my work and has become my friend.

In Texas, Ruth Poncik at Weimar Library has helped me find texts and has plied me with humor. Deborah Fitzpatrick, massage therapist, helped look after my body while I was looking after my soul. Betty Rainey and Dana Morrison, dear friends who with hugs and kind words soothed my soul and were patient with me when I was so engrossed in my work that I appeared to forget them. I never did—nor any of the other wonderful people who have shared my life.

And at Hodder & Stoughton, Laura Brockbank, my patient editor, who kept me on track and whose scribbled remarks so sweetly softened the blow of the cuts I had to make. Rowena Webb, Kerry Hood, Briar Silich, Anna Cade and all the team who had faith in me and rooted for this book to be born. The copyeditor, Beth Humphries, for her attention to detail and careful correction of the manuscript.

There are countless people who have helped me on my way and I ask their forgiveness that I haven't mentioned them. I give my heartfelt gratitude to all of those with whom I've had a privilege to work and acknowledge that I have been learning as well as teaching. And those who have taught me much in relationships that have shaped my life have held me in love even though there may be geographical distance between us.

My thanks and my love to you all.

Contents

Remember that where your heart is,
there is your treasure also.

—Foundation for Inner Peace,
A Course in Miracles

*T*his is a book about love: that fundamental vibration that stirs us to write poetry and sing songs, that leads each of us—fragments of a vast universe—to struggle to make sense of life and to come together and finally coalesce. That drives us to extend ourselves and become more than we ever thought possible. Love is an affinity that draws us towards each other and unites us in such a way that we feel complete and fulfilled. It is the only force which can join us at such a deep and fundamental level that it can completely change us and, indirectly, all of those with whom we come into contact whether or not we consciously desire this. In whatever form it presents itself—the sexual passion of lovers, the instinctual attachment of parents to their children, the loyalty which binds social groups and prompts men to die for their country, or the divine love that surpasses all human love and holds us as members of the body of the universe—love is the irresistible universal instinct that guides us all.

For some years I've struggled to find the semantics and terminology that feel right to me when trying to verbalize my thoughts and feelings about the Divine. Feeling instinctively that I needed to move beyond the restrictions of any particular religion, I used the term "the universe." This synthesis of human life, the planets including Earth, all life forms and all that fills the "space" between us, as well as the powerful cosmic affinity and love that flows through all, I see as a manifestation of the Divine. My own evolution has brought me to see the divine presence as the great soul of all souls; a great body of spirit from whence we all came. The term "God" seems once again more appropriate, and it is this that I've used here in the main. You may prefer to think in terms of a higher power, an infinite spirit, or to use your own name for that ultimate force. Whatever your understanding, whatever your preferred terminology, the force, the Divine, remains the same.

Though from time to time, and sometimes for long periods, we may feel lost and that our lives are not going in the direction we'd hoped, we are in fact following a purpose, some innate design that keeps us moving inexorably towards our reunion with God.

Those who are trying to make sense of life—to dot the i's and cross the t's and make things fit—lose the flow, the creativity and the enigma of life. In trying to pin down the mystery and make logic out of it, they lose the magic. For certainly, a kind of magic it is. In the same way as we are not only a collection of chemical equations, but also a soul, life itself is not only a series of events but a magical mystery tour; a treasure hunt with synchronicity and symbolism, signals and signposts urging us in the direction of easy progress. We can see with our hearts, feeling our way forward with integrity, or we can demand that life follows a pattern of our choosing, running the risk of missing all those enchanting byways that allow us unexpected discovery and unanticipated pleasure. Living from our hearts with love and intuition as the high road opens vistas of amazing beauty where we can linger and be nourished from the tips of our toes to the top of our soul. A literal, concrete viewpoint misses the lyrical and mystical quality that allows those with childlike simplicity, wisdom and vision to discern the authenticity and poetry of life. Open your heart, extend love to the universe, expect always the best and you will catch the gifts the universe is offering.

I really began to write this book twenty years ago or more when a simple transaction with someone I had never met changed my life.

While training as a psychiatrist in northeast England, I was on duty one night when an old man was brought in as an emergency admission. He'd been living under one of the bridges over the River Tyne and was frightened and disturbed. Though I'll talk more about him in Chapter 3, suffice to say here that he taught me much, including the true meaning of the wonderful greeting *"Namaste"*—"That part of God in me recognizes that part of God in you."

That transaction deepened my already profound conviction that love in all its manifestations can heal the wounds of the world. We should use with discrimination the best that modern technology has to offer—for that is a gift of God also. Few of us these days are meant to live a contemplative life in a monastery or up a mountain. I believe that we are called to action; to use all that we have to help heal—love being the major tool. The call of this new millennium is to make love visible in whatever way we can and to extend ourselves to share with each other the remarkable joy and peace that living in this way can produce. We can demonstrate a way of being that shuns violence, and we can at last move to a point of peace.

This book then is about a journey—an expedition through life as we learn again how to make that peace a reality. It's about relationships and relativity and how love in its various forms—or lack of it—affects everything. Everything affects everything else. Without understanding myself and my relationship with the various aspects of myself and with the rest of the universe, I feel lost, confused, out of control and sometimes afraid. Learning why I am where I am suddenly gives me focus and a sense of inner peace even though little may appear to have changed externally. This book will help you understand and accept where you are and why you're there and help you move on.

I talked about acceptance in *The 7 Healing Chakras* (Ulysses Press, 2000) and you may want to refer to that. But to recap, what I said was:

> Acceptance is a necessity before we can make
> a move that is well considered, understood,
> good for us and the next planned step on our
> journey through life.

If your goal is to understand more fully your present and future relationships then *Unlocking the Heart Chakra* can help you. An understanding and love of yourself is a great gift you can bring to any relationship. We must learn that we truly come into possession of ourselves when we allow ourselves to be lost in the love for another. Even the difficult parts of relationships can be embraced as spiritual experiences, making the whole more satisfying and fulfilling. Fun and excitement can replace pain and drama, though a little drama is like a touch of spice in your food: it gives a sweet, almost mystical lift, but too much spoils the flavor. Staying in line with your integrity helps you choose life partners who allow you to be who you really are and to be in a state of inner peace. Life without love is dry and tasteless, but with understanding and an open spiritual approach, it becomes a never-ending joyous feast. My wish for you as you begin is that you can experience love and life in all its glory.

All we need to do is to visualize our power of love developing until it encompasses all the universe.

One

How to Use This Book

*T*he plan is to focus on the love in your life—as it was, as it is and as it can become—and to heal yourself and the relationships that form the stuff of your daily life.

From birth and our relationship with parents, we move through the major connections in our lives to the point of divine love, which of course interlaces everything else. The emphasis is on healing, with love as our major tool, enabling us to move into a happier, healthier future with greater love and compassion for ourselves and others.

You may like to simply read through the book and then come back to issues you really want to work on, or you may like to work through bit by bit. It would be a good idea to have a notebook or journal to catch your thoughts and insights, write affirmations and map changes you make, and perhaps to jot down the odd quotation —not necessarily from this book, but from anything you read or hear. Sometimes when things are difficult, flipping through this and finding something that inspired you can lift your spirit and give you hope.

Try to write something every day. Just let your pen run across the page, your mind empty itself without stopping to analyze or correct what you've written. Do that later if you want to. You'll find that from time to time you slip into a different state, where your eyes feel a little blurry and your mind isn't engaged, but ideas are still pouring out on to the page. Try to let this continue without your mind getting in the way. Just let it flow. Your soul is talking! It will tell you truths you could neither have thought of nor worked out. Your life can be changed completely if you listen to, then act upon the messages you receive in that altered state.

Be gentle and compassionate with yourself and with the others in your life while everyone adjusts to the changes you're making.

Affirmations and Meditations

The affirmations I've chosen are simply a guide. Please change them into your own language. I remember well as a child reciting prayers in Sunday school and thinking that I just wanted to talk rather than say words that didn't feel right. Affirmations are a bit like that. After a while, new ones will simply start to come into your mind. Follow them and use them regularly, adjusting them word by word till they feel right for you.

Your subconscious mind takes things very literally, so you need to affirm in the present tense so that your subconscious will create things for you now rather than constantly keeping them in the future. Keep your affirmations simple and brief. Talk to your subconscious as you might talk to a child, giving simple instructions. If you'd like more affirmations, there's an address on page 303 from which you can order some.

The meditations are here just to guide you. You may find yourself wandering off into a meditation that comes from your spirit. As long as it's coming from a place of love, follow it—it will be far superior to anything I've written for you here. If you want to follow the meditations in the book exactly, that's fine—perhaps you could pre-record them onto a tape, or get a friend to read them for you as you relax.

You can meditate while walking but please don't do it in your car, though you can say your affirmations there! You'll gain more benefit if you make a special place for meditation. It doesn't have to be fancy or isolated—a particular chair will do—but if you can find a place where you won't be disturbed, where you can have a side table with a flower or two, a candle and a crystal, then that would be wonderful. Take the phone off the hook and give yourself time. Perhaps have some gentle music too. There are some suggestions at the end of this chapter. If you'd like a guided meditation, you might like to try my tape or CD, *Just Be*, which is available by mail order (see page 303).

After you have meditated, always allow yourself time to get properly grounded and close down your chakras before you resume your normal day. Have something to drink and perhaps a light snack; stretch a little or exercise gently.

Whatever you do, work gently. If you hit a difficult patch, breathe slowly and deeply, fill your heart with love and take time. The brief meditation on page 58 will help get you centered, grounded and back into the here and now.

Making Changes

Your life is your life; your relationships are your relationships; your choices are your choices. It's you and only you who can make changes in your life. But you can't change anyone else. I'm afraid that if you're unhappy, the only person who can do something about it is you.

I often hear people lament, "But I've done all the changing!" Well, sometimes it feels that way, but if you're still not happy with your lot, it sounds as though there's still changing to do. Every shift you make within yourself will result in some change within relationships whether or not that was your intention. At times we make changes and the result isn't what we wanted at all, but that means that we just have to modify things again. In general, changes need to be small, giving time for you and those in your life to adjust so you can see the result before you make another change.

Sometimes, however, you just *know* that you need to alter things radically. If for instance there's violence between you and your partner, or involving children, something radical needs to happen now. If there's drinking or drug taking that's draining you of your self-esteem, self-confidence and peace of mind, something needs to happen now. If you're chronically unhappy, then you need to look at why. And if you feel depressed, you may need some professional help. There's a quick checklist in Appendix 3 (page 298) to help you decide what you might need.

Learning to listen to all of yourself—body, mind and soul— will help you know what you need. Meditating and allowing stresses to surface and heal will help too. Having someone you can trust to talk to, to cry with or be angry with, and know they won't run away, is a great gift while you're making changes. A good therapist should be able to offer you all of that and gently reflect to you what appears to be going on. She won't tell you what to do, but will help you decide for yourself where to go next. Sometimes clients say to me, "Please help me," missing the fact that in listening with empathy, compassion and an open heart, I'm already doing so by giving them space to help themselves. But if your resources are so depleted that you feel you can't make decisions for yourself, perhaps you need to decide to make no decisions right now. That's okay: you'll be gathering strength to move when the time is right. But try not to stay in that place for too long. When you eventually make a move, I assure

---

A word of caution and encouragement . . .

We're human beings and for most of us, no matter how enlightened we become, there'll be challenges in life that disturb us from time to time. These may be relationships we've chosen to help us discover more about ourselves, or the plight of people in parts of the world where there is abject poverty, natural disasters or the corruption that seems to be an integral part of the fabric of politics. Don't be distressed if you find that despite spiritual practice and trying your very best to live in love and harmony, you still find yourself being angry, gossiping or staying in abusive situations you know you should leave.

Be gentle with yourself and don't use what you see as failure as an excuse to give up on yourself. Look at what you are learning from being where you are, and gently make whatever changes you need to make. Occasionally these may be huge, radical changes, but more often we need to take baby steps towards our true spiritual self and peace. Eventually we will reach a place of balance and harmony where we can observe with compassion and yet not feel the agony. In non-attachment we can be free.

---

you, you'll be supported—whether by friends, your family, your partner or God—every inch of the way. Try to trust.

I hope your changes will be joyful, but of course there may be painful and difficult times on the way. Even if you can't make an external change, for example you can't leave because you have no financial support and nowhere else to go, an inner change can be empowering and will automatically render those around you powerless to hold you hostage. Your mind and your soul can never be imprisoned. But do make sure that the power you use to empower yourself is never used negatively towards anyone else. The knowledge you gain on your journey is yours, and though you may wish to share, try not to be too evangelical since this can alienate people. As you change you'll be amazed at how everyone else does too. But let them find their own time.

Always try to keep focused on the moment. Savoring each instant, even the painful ones, helps us to learn and move along more quickly.

And try to keep your sense of humor! Difficult if you're feeling pain. But sometimes humor can effect change like nothing else. Keep things light and simple and you'll be surprised at what can happen.

Detachment from the Outcome

Please work through the whole book without preconceived ideas, if possible. Even if you have no siblings, for instance, the chapter on brothers and sisters will help you understand and deepen the connection with those in your life who do.

If you decided in the past that your only recourse was to detach from someone, whether parent, brother or sister, friend or partner, then there are still things for you both to learn. Though you may have detached here on this plane, a connection will always exist between you. Send them light and let them be.

In reading this book you may be preparing to heal both yourself and relationships that have been difficult, and from a new perspective breathe life and love into those relationships again, in neither a patronizing nor a superior way, but with a desire that whatever happens will be for the higher good of you both. Even if you have to approach the relationship from a distance and without direct contact, the healing can touch both of you and bring resolution to old wounds and trauma. Even if you never see the person again, you can achieve a place of peace for yourself. You deserve that.

Choose carefully whom you share your journey with. You may want to be a bit secretive and protective of what you're discovering

---

Music Suggestions

Music for Healing, *Stephen Rhodes, New World Music*
Gracefully, *Giovanni Marradi, Newcastle Entertainment*
The Elegance of Pachelbel, *Michael Maxwell, Avalon Music*

---

and feeling. On the other hand, you may want to shout from the rooftops when you have some glorious insight. That's not usually the best thing to do. Others may rain on your parade and put doubt into your mind about the veracity of what you've found before you've had time to completely integrate it. Stay with your own truth. It will serve you well. You'll soon learn to recognize a true insight because you'll feel an excitement in your heart, sudden clarity, and ideas will flow. Insight is always accompanied by love, because that's all your soul knows.

Have a wonderful journey. Wherever you're going, it's a privilege to be part of your path in this moment. I wish you joy, good companionship, laughter and the help of angels. Fill yourself with love and connect with your heart and soul. The very fact that you're reading this says that there's a link between us. Down that connection, through time and space, I send you love.

Meditation

Meditating, praying and asking for guidance in whatever way you prefer can go a long way to setting you free. At hard times in my life I'd often simply say, "Please show me the way." And the way would eventually become clear. Watch for synchronicity—those hints from the universe about the path you're to take. If you keep your eyes open and your senses alert, the universe will lead you out of even the most difficult places. And constantly give thanks for where you are. That might sound crazy when you're in a painful place. But if you can approach it with genuine gratitude so that whatever you're supposed to be gaining from it you can absorb right now, your days in that wilderness will be numbered.

Two

The Energy System
❧

Truth is within ourselves; it takes no rise
From outward things, whate'er you may believe:
There is an inmost center in us all,
Where truth abides in fulness.

—ROBERT BROWNING, "PARACELSUS," I

ove is an amazing force that has roots in every bit of us, flowing throughout our whole being, a many-faceted divine gift we can use to heal, to comfort, to move mountains. Our capacity to love develops throughout our lives, and depends to a large extent on the health and evolvement of our inner energy system. If we've suffered trauma that has left us feeling bitter, controlling or unable to feel tenderness, then healthy loving becomes a minefield where games are played and people get hurt. (If you've suffered a life event that has severely disturbed you, such as some form of abuse or a loss for which you're still grieving, now might be the time to find a good therapist.) Problems at one level lead to difficulties at others, since the free flow of energy is blocked, leading to distortions further up or down the system. Understanding this helps us to clear the problems we've developed and frees us to learn to love ourselves and others with our hearts and souls and to allow others to love us appropriately too.

Should you want to look at your energy system in more detail, my book *The 7 Healing Chakras* will help you.

This chapter gives an overall view of the topography of the energy system, with suggestions for working on each center and also an affirmation that will help. If you feel a chakra (see page 20) is in difficulty, try wearing something of the color of that center—a handkerchief or a scarf will do, or something worn under your clothes. At the end of the chapter is a meditation for balancing your energy system and bringing your chakras into alignment.

To understand love as a dynamic energy that you can utilize and direct as well as feel, it's essential to grasp the structure of your energetic system and how it works. You can learn to feel your energy as it flows or gets stuck, and though it may take some practice, eventually you'll be able to create inner peace as you come into harmony and balance. Your energy will tell you very accurately when things you're doing are not in line with your integrity, when you need to get back on track; it will give you the courage to reverse decisions, to do things differently, stand up for what you know is right and direct your life in a more conscious way. You will know very clearly what's right for you, regardless of what might appear right for others. Intuitively you will be more aware of the real message behind other people's behavior also.

Energy

Energy is the stuff of which everything is made. The universe is a massive energy system—particles vibrating at various frequencies making up all there is, and that includes us. The molecules that make up my body, and yours, are formed from the same elements that make everything else—plants and animals, the chair you're sitting on and the air we breathe. The only difference is in the combination of the particles and the frequency with which they vibrate. Depending upon the vibrational frequency, some things appear more dense than others. Solids have densely packed fast-moving molecules whereas gases, which have molecules moving more slowly, are less dense and appear very different. This results in some things being visible and others not. Being invisible to the human eye doesn't make things less real—think of radio and TV waves and electric currents for instance.

Sometimes part of something is visible and part is not. Your television set is visible but the waves that form the picture aren't until they're caught on the screen. The same is true of your body. There's a dense part, the physical body, which we usually think of as being our total body. But around it there's another part of our body that is invisible to most people, though some healers and mystics can see it clearly. In fact, if we were to think of it correctly, we'd see that the physical body is the bit inside the whole body, the outside being just as real, rather like a fruit with a seed—the harder, denser piece is in the middle.

Universal Energy Field (UEF)

Sometimes simply termed "the field," this is the matrix that connects us all. It's the "space" between the solid, liquid and gas objects of which we're generally aware, and contains light rays, sound waves, television and radio signals as well as the air we breathe and various other forms of energy. It holds energy emitted by the stars, the planets and other celestial bodies as well as whatever dwells in the vast universe. It is, as its name implies, the energy of the universe.

Since everything is made of moving energy, the UEF is constantly in motion, not only because of the winds and air streams that surround the planet, but also because of the vibrational field set up by everything.

We can change the energy in the field by what we do, think, feel, say, how we move and what quality of energy we emit. Thus we're all responsible for whether the field remains calm and peaceful or becomes turbulent and uneasy. What happens in the field affects us just as we affect it. Just think what happens when you walk into a room: what you smell, what you see, the colors and how people talk to you and behave towards you make you feel different. In fact they bring about neurological changes within you as a direct result of the energy flowing in the field and into you. If you change your external environment, by walking on the beach for instance, you'll have a different kind of energy flowing around and into you, and your internal environment changes.

We can learn to manipulate the field by controlling our feelings, by sending out loving energy and by behaving in a calm and serene manner. We can also disturb it and the people in it by emitting harsh, prickly vibrations. Thus we have a responsibility to be aware of what we're doing when we behave badly. Not only will you and the people within your part of the field be affected, but the vibrations will go on for ever, affecting a wider and wider circle of people. We'll discuss this in more detail in Chapter 9.

Your Aura or Human Energy Field

Though you may not realize it, you've been subjected to pictures of the human energy field every time you've seen a stained-glass window in a church which depicts Christ or one of the saints. The halo around the heads of these figures, and the light that appears to be emitted by them, is their aura. This is the outer part of our body we referred to earlier. Your aura is your soul light, which displays around you much of who you are and how you feel. Sometimes it's referred to as the subtle body or bodies, since it contains several layers that all have different functions. It's present in everyone, though in some people it's very bright and clear and in others it appears to be smaller and less bright though not necessarily less powerful.

The aura is full of things—just as wonderful as the inner workings of your physical body. It also has several functions. First of all it's your personal space. If someone steps too close and enters into your aura without being invited to do so, you may feel quite uncomfortable and take a step back. It helps us negotiate the outside world and since it precedes us, it senses things before our physical body does. It has a protective function, filtering out much of what goes on around us so that we're neither bombarded nor flooded with energy from elsewhere. Sometimes it fails in this function and we do feel swamped as other people's energy gets mixed up with ours. Our aura also generally protects us to some degree from psychic pollution. Unfortunately, since so many people are unaware that they even have an aura, they don't take care of it and it can get damaged and dirty.

Your aura can be cleansed very simply (see page 35) and damage can be healed.

Sensing with Your Aura

We generally accept that we sense the world around us with touch, sight, hearing, smell and taste. The aura helps us sense the world in a different way, since when finely tuned, it can pick up subtle changes in atmosphere, changes in the moods of those around us and the nuances of energy when they feel uncomfortable: when, for example, they're not telling the truth. We can detect very quickly if something enters our energy field that changes it and the aura also tells us what we're emitting into the world around us. A finely tuned aura refines our perception as we monitor the space in which we live, rather like having a personal radar which detects shifts in our own and other people's consciousness and gives us information that is otherwise unavailable to us. Some people would refer to this broadly as intuition, though intuition is only a small part of the process of sensing with your energy body.

Other sensitive people can pick up similar information about us, so it's a good idea to be responsible and self-aware, trying to ensure that what we emit into the world is peaceful and harmonious.

Every single transaction we have with another human being (and also with other things) includes an exchange of energy. It's up to you what kind of energy exchange you want to have. If you want to remain peaceful, then steer clear of those who are emitting angry clouds and flashes of energy that either hang in your space or cut into your aura like knives. With some people you feel that your energy gets sucked out, leaving you feeling tired, drained and low in both energy and mood. Be more aware next time you see such a person. If you could see the energy flow, you would observe your aura becoming depleted while your energy is being taken into the other person's energy body and they start to feel better. Sadly, many people take others' energy quite unconsciously, but if you're to continue seeing them you need to learn to protect yourself (see page 35).

Just as some people have an aura which feels uncomfortable to others, others carry with them peace, serenity and love that is tangible to everyone who meets them. These people are usually very aware. They spend time meditating or praying or actively thinking positive thoughts, making their aura sparkling and bright. They touch every other aura with which they come into contact, brightening it and spreading inspiration. In their presence you feel energized and are happy to see them: you want to spend time with them because they infect their contacts with joy.

As your auric sense becomes more acute, please be discreet and don't intrude into other people's privacy.

Take a moment and imagine what it must be like being around you. Are you emitting peace and happiness, lightness and joy? Do you feel full of energy yourself, and is your mood sunny? Or are you heavy and critical, suspicious of others and judgmental of what they do? What kind of atmosphere do you think that will bring when you enter a room? Will people be happy to be around you or does your energy drag them down?

It may be that you feel depressed or that there's little love in your life. Don't be hard on yourself if you have to answer that in all honesty your energy may not be very pleasant to be around. There's lots you can do about that as you move through the book, and just being aware of it helps. Try to see the good things about people, smile when you meet someone, share a pleasantry with the person at the checkout or just say "good morning" to someone on the street and your energy will start to shift and you, and those around you, will start to feel better. And if you can see that your energy isn't good because of the people you're usually with, then look at whether you want to change that. If you're living with someone who's depressed or ill, make sure you get out and have some fun, which will help keep your own energy in balance.

The best way to clear your aura and make it sparkle is to have love in your heart. That doesn't mean necessarily being in love, but *feeling* love. And clearing up the mess that causes us to feel dull and lifeless or downright miserable. Doing what you love and loving what you do can make a great difference to the energy of your aura, which in turn nurtures your physical body and touches everyone around you.

Grounding

Before we talk about the intricate energy system within the aura, let's look for a moment at the phenomenon of grounding.

We're spiritual beings occupying human bodies, and we need to stay rooted in the earth to accomplish all we came here to do. However, it's easy for a split to occur between your spiritual and physical self. Your soul can become displaced, leaving you feeling outside of yourself, as though you're floating above the ground as an observer. Sometimes during a traumatic incident we experience this phenomenon, known as "dissociation." Usually we later re-enter our body, but in some cases people stay separated from their bodies for years. For some, dissociation becomes a habit whenever anything threatens them. Some people haven't wanted to come to earth at all and have never fully occupied their bodies. After meditating or witnessing something inspiring and uplifting, we might not want to come back to everyday life and don't quite get "grounded"; this leaves us appearing somewhat preoccupied and strange.

In all of these cases, the answer is grounding. In fact grounding should be part of one's daily routine and certainly should follow any meditation. The process is very simple. Going for a walk, eating or drinking or doing breathing exercises will help ground you. Food, particularly thick hearty soups and porridge, are grounding. Dancing, especially to music with a real beat, will attach you to the earth, as will gardening or working with clay. There are also specific grounding exercises. One can be found at the end of this chapter and others are given in more detail in *The 7 Healing Chakras*.

Our aim in grounding is to connect with the earth while remaining in our body, in our consciousness in the here and now. This allows us to be acutely aware of our own movements and surroundings, and helps us to feel rooted, strong and able to cope with difficulties.

The Chakra System

Within the aura are countless sensory communication points and also a well-organized sensory system—the chakra system. Chakras are communication centers—wheels of light which, when in good health, are constantly spinning, drawing in energy from the UEF, revitalizing our whole system and emitting energy too.

Psychic pollution and psychic attack

Psychic pollution is very common; active psychic attack less so. Both need to be taken seriously if you are to protect your energy and take care of that part of your body that is your aura.

Some people simply have bad energy caused by something that happened to them long ago and left them wounded and with a tendency to behave in a manner that isn't conducive to peace.

If you find that suddenly your self-confidence falls, you start to feel self-doubt, fear, despair or negativity that is foreign to you, if you are scapegoated or witness that happening to someone else, then it's worth thinking of psychic pollution and possibly psychic attack. Sometimes psychic attack will render you weak and depressed and makes you feel as though things are happening to you that you don't understand.

Often the cause is that someone is directing bad energy towards you—not necessarily consciously—and you need to protect yourself. See the protection exercise on page 35. Remember that no one has any real power over you and that negative energy is never as strong as positive energy. Though you may have been caught unaware (and that happens to all of us sometimes), you can get yourself back in balance quite quickly if you work on it.

The major chakras are arranged in a vertical line from below the base of the spine to above the crown of the head and each spins at a specific frequency. Each has its own morphology and set of functions; they're all different colors, depending on the frequency of their vibration and their state of health. The lowest, the root or base chakra, is red and the others, in ascending order, bear the other colors of the spectrum—orange, yellow, green, blue, indigo and purple or white. They're numbered from the bottom upwards.

These are the extrasensory organs, which relay information to us about others and to others about us. The information they can give us is extremely accurate. We'll be discussing the seven major ones here. There are also 21 minor ones and many lesser ones situated at acupuncture points. Each of the chakras is associated with a particular layer of the aura—the first with the layer closest to the solid physical body, the second with the next one, and so on. The specific layers of the aura are difficult to see and the whole is more likely to be perceived as a shimmering mass with some areas of different color and consistency within it.

Each chakra is like a spiraling trumpet extending from the physical body through the aura to the outside where it communicates with the UEF. Each has petals and, like a sea anemone, it can gently open and close, filtering the energy that can come and go. Sometimes chakras become stagnant, the flow of energy blocked, or they may be wide open and stiff, their ability to filter and protect lost. Sometimes they become physically damaged or torn. The term "a broken heart" has some substance if we look at the heart chakra: the heart bond we've made with another is wrenched free as the person dies or leaves us, rendering the chakra unable to function properly till it heals. The solar plexus often has the same problem after the sudden loss of a loved one since the bonds formed there are torn too. The powerlessness and weakness often associated with grief are in part caused by these wounds to the energy system, which may take a long time to heal.

Each chakra is also associated with a major gland and nerve plexus. I'll mention these briefly as we look at the chakras individually.

Though all the chakras are present in a fairly rudimentary form when we're born, they continue to develop and refine as we grow. The first, the root chakra, develops between birth and the age of three to five. Next is the sacral, developing between three to five and eight years old and, following this, the solar plexus between the age of eight and twelve. These lower three chakras deal with the physical, and damage to them as they're developing causes us problems in relating to the world. This will be discussed in detail later. The heart chakra develops between 12 and 16 and is a transitional chakra bridging the gap between the physical and the spiritual world. Next the throat, which develops at 16 to 21, the brow at 21 to 26, and finally the crown. Though the upper chakras may never develop much within a lifetime, the rewards are great for those who are willing to work on them.

Each chakra can be seen as a plane of consciousness, one building upon another until the spiritual personality is fully developed. Various spiritual gifts such as healing and clairvoyance develop simultaneously. Sometimes there's a precocious development. After the age of about 30, when the chakra system has naturally developed along with our physical body, we start to refine it. People may spontaneously want to revisit their roots and make considerable changes in their lives between the ages of 28 and 31 and look at relationships and their sexuality again between about 33 and 38. Often we can work out, albeit roughly, the kind of issues people will be dealing with at various times in their lives. From the way we behave it's also easy to see when there was earlier trauma, since the natural chakra development has been arrested or distorted in some way, preventing us from interpreting life with the maturity one would expect.

Though this may seem academic, it becomes very practical both in studying ourselves and others in our lives, and in being aware of the issues our children and others may be facing at various ages. Though the chapters that follow may make little reference to the chakras, a basic knowledge can add excitement as we understand ourselves more and see that our past leads us to behave in certain ways. If you wish to know more about your energy system, *The 7 Healing Chakras* deals with it in much greater detail. The next chapter will talk more about the heart chakra, since its energy and love affects every area of our lives.

So let's have a quick overview of the chakras.

THE ROOT OR BASE CHAKRA

This is the first chakra to develop and is situated at the perineum, that bit of tissue between the vagina or scrotum and anus. It spins more slowly than the others (at the speed of red light), roots us to the planet and deals with basic instincts and survival. It prompts us to take care of ourselves, governing such essential activities as eating, sleeping and procreation. If it had a voice, it would say "I am."

If there's trauma during its natural development, for example maternal separation or illness that threatens the security of the child, the root chakra fails to develop properly. It might be underactive or overactive—in either case basic instincts and the will to survive are affected. Underactivity generally causes ambivalence about caring for ourselves and even being alive. We have poor eating and sleeping habits and can be apathetic or depressed. Sometimes such people take risks with their lives, for example by following dangerous sports or not taking common safety precautions. They may have an unconscious desire to leave the planet, and may use alcohol or drugs to help them dissociate, if only temporarily. Sometimes they actively want to die and may attempt suicide. If the chakra is overactive they're over-concerned about survival, fearing that something is going to happen to them, being defensive and perceiving slight and attack where there is none. Men may have sexual problems such as erectile dysfunction and women are usually unable to have an orgasm.

The root chakra governs the adrenal glands, which produce and secrete steroids, and is associated with the coccygeal nerve plexus, which supplies the genital region.

Getting the root chakra in balance demands that we do some work to improve our feeling of being rooted to the planet. Walks in the country or on the beach, resting when we're tired and eating when we're hungry can help. Many people with root chakra problems wander about, move house every few years and never seem to feel at home anywhere despite a honeymoon phase in each new place they move to. Balancing your root chakra will bring you great rewards: You will feel comfortable and happy to be alive and will have a sense of belonging. Women will start to put their own needs higher up the list.

A good affirmation for the root chakra is: *I am part of the earth and the vast cosmos and I am happy to be alive. My life is a gift to me and to all of humanity.*

THE SACRAL CHAKRA

This chakra can be found in the lower abdomen and is fiery orange in color. It governs our sexuality—quite different from the basic sexual instinct of the root chakra. It also governs the pleasure/pain principle and sensuality, and the giving and receiving of sexual pleasure. The sacral chakra prompts us to start to relate to others and to reach out to the world. The inner balance of our masculine and feminine principles (see also Chapter 8) begins here. Creativity also starts to develop here. The sacral is an emotional chakra and, governed by water, helps us to be flexible and flowing, to perceive beauty around us and "go with the flow." If it could talk, it would say "I feel."

If it is overactive there can be an insatiable desire for pleasure, often of a sexual kind, leading to a hedonistic life that can never fill the void within. Underactivity leads to disinterest in life, rigidity, depression and lack of desire. Sensual pleasure just doesn't exist for people with a sacral block, and creative expression is low.

The sacral chakra governs the ovaries in women and the testicles in men. It's associated with the sacral nerve plexus supplying the buttocks, thighs and lower limbs.

Balance can be achieved by dealing with whatever trauma occurred at the age when it was developing (roughly five to eight) and by visualizing the color orange in the region below the navel. Rituals involving water, such as taking long luxurious baths, standing in the shower meditating, swimming or sitting under a waterfall will help.

A good affirmation for the sacral chakra is: *I am flexible and flowing in harmony with the universe. My creativity flows forth to enhance my life and that of others.*

THE SOLAR PLEXUS CHAKRA

This powerful chakra is in the upper abdomen, sometimes slightly to the left. It shines bright yellow like the midday sun and is your personal power center. Here your will develops and hence your willpower, decisions and opinions. It's also the place of prosperity. With a healthy solar plexus we're committed to meeting our own needs, to getting what we really want, and we move along a path that we know is right for us. It's the center of the mind and if it could talk, it would say "I will."

Because it encompasses our will and power, if it's blocked, unhealthy or out of balance we can be weak-willed, passive and easily led, with little opinion of our own, a lack of commitment and an inability to find our own path. If your solar plexus is overactive, then you're likely to be bossy and domineering, unaware that your power can hurt others if misused. We need to remind ourselves that we're blessed with power to do things and must not overpower others. Bullying, meddling, controlling others and telling them how to live their lives are hallmarks of the overstimulated solar plexus chakra. If you or someone you know is like that, then the root often lies in what was happening to them around the ages of eight to twelve when this powerhouse was developing.

The solar plexus is associated with the pancreas, which secretes insulin and glucagon, both essential for carbohydrate metabolism.

Getting the solar plexus in balance demands that we address our power and ensure that we use it wisely and well. Enjoy it, revel in it, but never use it against anyone. We have a duty to take control of our own lives, but never those of others since we have no idea where they're going or what path they need to take. That includes our children. We'll discuss this more in Chapter 5. Spend some time in the sun (wearing a sunscreen, of course) and draw into yourself the power of the universe, allowing it to fill every part of you with golden yellow light.

A good affirmation for the solar plexus is: *I am balanced and in control of my own life. I have the power to live well and to make choices that are right for me.*

THE HEART CHAKRA

The whole of the next chapter is about the heart chakra so I won't discuss it extensively here.

It's associated with the thymus gland and the pulmonary and cardiac nerve plexuses, which are really an extension of each other and supply the respiratory tract, the heart, the aorta and the pulmonary vein.

A good affirmation for the heart chakra is: *I open to give and receive love. I love myself and all those around me.*

THE THROAT CHAKRA

The throat chakra is situated at the base of your neck, a little higher at the back of the neck than the front (unlike the other chakras, which are found at the same level back and front). It's the azure blue of the sky or sometimes slightly turquoise. The throat chakra puts out into the world that creativity that began at the sacral, the decisions and opinions we started to develop in the solar plexus and the love we feel in our hearts. It encompasses communication in all its forms, building on the levels of consciousness we've already developed on our ascent. There's little point in being clear of voice if we have nothing to say, no opinion to express. But the throat chakra prompts us to go further. It urges us to speak our truth, to have the courage to stand up for what we believe and take action.

Right now, I'm using my throat chakra to pull together the messages of my other chakras and communicate them to you, albeit in writing. The essence of my truth, my opinions, my experience, my love, my visions, my understanding, is being made known via my throat chakra. It also encompasses my integrity and my vocation.

A well-balanced throat chakra enables us to make a difference in the world by expressing ourselves with clarity. People usually listen to what comes from a healthy throat chakra since it has a ring of truth that is unmistakable.

A throat chakra that is out of balance makes it difficult for us to sort out what we really want to say, and our message becomes confused and gets lost. People with a blocked or underdeveloped throat often talk *at* others rather than *to* them, or are wordy but say nothing. Sometimes they actively lie, though often this is because they don't really know what they think or what the truth of the matter is. They have a lot of conflicting mind chatter that impedes clarity of thought, slows them down and makes articulation difficult. Sometimes it causes them to become passive and blend into the wallpaper, apparently having nothing to contribute. Sometimes they become angry and aggressive in their speech while really making little sense.

The throat chakra is associated with the thyroid and parathyroid glands, which affect metabolism, growth, temperature control, energy production and carbohydrate and fat metabolism. It's also connected with the pharyngeal plexus supplying the pharynx and tongue and the brachial plexus, which supplies the arms.

Visualizing a blue light at your throat will help clear and balance this chakra, as will using your voice in a pleasant manner. Singing, chanting, praying, toning (sounding a continuous note) and speaking (alone at first if you feel shy and need to build confidence) will help. Consciously listening, being truthful (kindly) and paying attention to what you say will clarify your communication. Thinking and then speaking rather than blurting out a reaction will also help. As always, the more you practice, the better it will be. Look forward to the time when you can speak with command, can caress with gentle words, can stand against the crowd if your truth and integrity differ from their's, can be self-assertive in conflict and not participate when insults get thrown around. Communication in other forms such as writing, keeping a diary or playing an instrument; being creative and expressing yourself in painting, pottery, movement, dance, whatever —will help you open to the vast area of your creative expression that you may never have thought possible. Just keep focused on your throat and let the message of your soul pour forth.

The spiritual gifts of this chakra are clairaudience and telepathy. It's here that we often start to hear messages from our guides and helpers, though for some this never happens—and that's fine.

If the throat chakra could speak it would say "I communicate, I hear."

A good affirmation is: *I speak my truth to the whole world with love, gentleness, integrity and faith. I am open to receive the messages of the universe that pour into me now.*

THE BROW CHAKRA

Above and between our eyes, the brow chakra—sometimes erroneously called the third eye—helps us see the whole world through spiritual eyes. The color here is deep blue, sometimes as deep as indigo and sometimes the color of lapis lazuli or even tinged with purple.

This is the center of vision, but not merely of physical sight. We can see with clarity that everything is absolutely in its rightful place as part of an amazing pattern and the beauty of everything becomes visible. Usually we interpret visual stimuli as they fall on our retina. Through the brow chakra we can see even if we're physically blind. On an inner screen we can play out an array of scenes—past, present and future—in a moment. It's also the place of imagination and daydreaming and is where our dreams show us the inner workings of our subconscious, in a symbolic way. Though we have raw intuition in our solar plexus (our gut feelings), it's here that our intuition is perfected and we have at our fingertips another highly accurate sense. The spiritual gift is clairvoyance.

If the brow chakra is overstimulated and overactive, imaginings and dreams appear to become reality, and various psychiatric disorders can develop, with hallucinations and delusions causing great confusion. Some drugs such as Ecstasy, cannabis and cocaine may overstimulate this chakra and cause permanent damage. When blocked there is little "imagination," and we have difficulty in visualizing and in feeling inspired.

Visualizing deep blue light emitting from your forehead and looking down its beam, imagining what you can see, will help develop or restore this chakra to health. Don't worry that you might be "making up" what you see. Just relax and let anything flow into your mind, trusting that whatever it is, it has some kind of meaning for you even if you don't recognize it right now. Why not jot down in your journal what you "see," no matter how disjointed or trivial it seems. You may be surprised to come back to it later and find that it did have meaning. The more you check it out, the more you'll be able to allow yourself to trust your new-found skill. Looking at things through spiritual eyes, you see much more of the picture. If your world seems clouded by pain and negativity, the chances are you're missing some of the joy and beauty that could be coming your way. This chakra sometimes doesn't develop in a lifetime, so don't worry if yours hasn't.

The brow chakra is associated with the pineal gland, though some would claim it is attached to the pituitary and hypothalamus. The pineal secretes melatonin and governs sleep by monitoring our body clock. It may also have some effect on ageing and sexual function. Its nervous connection is to the carotid plexus, which supplies the head, neck and ears.

If it could talk, the brow chakra would say, "I see."

A good affirmation is: *I see the world with spiritual eyes and perceive the truth and beauty in all things.*

THE CROWN CHAKRA

At the top and slightly above your head is your crown chakra, glowing with a deep purple or white light. Here is your access to the divine, the site where your soul enters your physical body. Here, at the center of knowing, we can draw in divine energy to augment our own and use it to heal ourselves and others. Here we find ourselves beyond understanding, intellectual discussion or reason, in a place of indescribable knowing. Messages that enter here can be trusted, but make sure your ego is out of the way and you're not thinking. The sensation is quite different.

Here is your path, your soul's purpose, your calm awareness and certainty about who you are and why you came here, of where you should go and what you should do. The messages that come in at your crown transcend all others. It just *is*. We all have flashes of this awareness from time to time—often when there's some crisis in our lives and suddenly we know what to do and how to do it in a way that's beyond our usual understanding. Such flashes of knowing may completely change our lives or the lives of others, and then leave us once again very normal human beings, as amazed as everyone else about what we did and how we did it, though often with a profound new sense of well-being. Here, at our crown, our soul speaks to us, our spirit connects with the body of God and we can hear the divine call our name.

The crown chakra, associated with the pituitary gland, which is the grand regulator of the whole endocrine system and with the cerebral cortex, which commands everything, says "I know." The gift of the crown is channeling, where you stand aside, suspend judgement and criticism and are open to allow wisdom to enter, unfettered. If you try to listen and to think about what's happening, you'll lose the connection and hit the earth with a thud. The messages that come from the divine may be different from what we expected and may even oppose our own opinions.

Often the crown doesn't develop in an earthly lifetime. But the fact that you're reading this indicates that you're on a developmental journey and that this is a possibility for you. *The 7 Healing Chakras* has meditations for the crown chakra and we'll also revisit it in Chapter 10.

Building on the Foundations

As you see, each chakra has its foundation in the one below. And so it is with life. Each of our experiences builds on the ones before and we put into practice in one relationship what we have learned in previous ones. It's the relationships with our primary careers, hopefully our parents, which set us on course for all other relationships. And relationships with siblings add their input as we later choose friends and partners, and so on. Thus how we behave with colleagues at work may well be due to how we perceived an elder sister, and the person we choose to marry is not only influenced by the kind of father we had, but also by the way the teacher treated us at school and how that reflected bullying by a brother. All are intertwined. And all can be changed and healed if we work through what has happened to us on our journey through life thus far. So by understanding and healing our past relationships we can stop repeating mistakes that our parents made with us and that we've been making too. This can help us see our life partners as who they are rather than whom we want them to be and to appreciate their beauty or decide to leave. It can help us stop seeing that colleague at work as the mother who constantly told us what to wear and how to behave and never gave us credit for having a brain in our heads, and can even help us see the love and care that was behind that behavior.

Life is all about experiencing as much as we can and rendering ourselves more whole in the process. But if we continue to wear blinders and refuse to broaden our view, then our lives become narrow, sad and painful.

The next chapter will help you look more closely at your heart and the hearts of others and then put that into the context of the relationships that have shaped your life. It will help you see the truth behind illusions and help you decide upon your direction. You have all that you need to orientate your life perfectly and live as the spiritual being you are, with love for yourself and all the universe.

Enjoy your journey.

Exercises

GROUNDING

Grounding can be as easy as breathing and helps you to stay in the moment. You can dance to music with a good beat, have a bath with a handful of Epsom salts in the water, exercise and experience your body, hold a crystal. However, if you like ritual, here's a simple grounding exercise.

If you can do this outside with your shoes off, great; but since spiritual energy can get from here to the other side of the earth, it can surely get through the soles of your shoes and into the earth even if you're on the tenth floor. So don't worry about that.

Stand or sit with your feet a little distance apart. If for some reason you either can't stand or can't sit, it doesn't matter. Just imagine yourself doing so. Close your eyes and imagine roots going down from the soles of your feet and your open root chakra deep into the earth, holding you like a tree, strong and straight. Imagine now that you are drawing up the golden energy of the earth through those roots, healing, nurturing, strong and empowering, up through your legs and into the base of your pelvis. Feel it warming you, filling you with earthy energy. Know that you are part of the earth, that you belong here and the earth will make you strong.

Now allow that energy to come right up to the level of your heart and flow into and around your heart, strong and protective. Hold it there, a golden ball surrounding and filling your heart.

If you can, lift your arms up now, hands upturned to the sky, and allow the energy of the universe to come streaming down into your hands and the top of your head, silver white light, streaming in and filling your head and upper body. Let it come down to the level of your heart where it mingles with the wonderful golden energy of the earth. The energy of all that exists is flowing through you now. Let the silver and the gold combine and fill every part of you. Feel yourself nourished and strengthened. Breathe slowly and deeply and allow yourself to enjoy the power that fills you.

Take your hands now and cup them around your heart. Affirm your being. Affirm your belonging. Allow yourself to just be.

Stay as long as you wish. When you're ready, withdraw the roots from the earth while knowing that you remain rooted in this lifetime, your physical body a part of the earth. Feel yourself grounded. Stretch. Move a little. Have a drink of water and take your time before getting on with your day.

CLEANSING AND PROTECTION

You can cleanse and protect yourself with a thought, but it's nice to bring the whole thing to awareness and enjoy what you're doing. Any ritual involving water will do: a bath, shower, stream, waterfall or even standing outside on a sunny afternoon and running water from the garden hose over you while consciously intending to cleanse your aura. You can do the same thing in your imagination.

If you prefer a ritual, you might like to try the following, which I particularly love to do. I like to have the house completely to myself and I have a white caftan (though anything will do) that I put on afterwards, even if only for a while. A soft white towel or a blanket would do just as well, or even snuggling down into clean sheets.

First of all I like to prepare myself by spending a moment thinking about where I am and what energy around me is mine and what belongs to other people. What have I picked up during the day and want to let go of? What have I felt uncomfortable or angry about that I want to cleanse myself of now? Has anyone been clinging to me and leaving parts of themselves around me? Have I done the same thing?

I then set my intention to heal, and close my eyes. I call to any part of myself that may have gotten displaced during the day to come home and lovingly join with me. I also lovingly ask that anything that does not belong with me should return to whence it came. I visualize myself as whole, my aura smooth and intact.

I open my chakras one by one by visualizing them spinning faster and opening till I can see all the colors like gems in my aura. Don't worry if you can't do this immediately. With practice it will come. Finally I open my crown and ask that the highest possible light and love will flow into me, cleanse me, balance me, heal me and protect me, and I just allow the energy to flow. Sometimes I feel so humble at this point that tears stream down my face. Sometimes I feel so powerful that my head lifts up my face to the heavens and I know that I'm glowing.

I then ask that all that needs to be forgiven is forgiven, that my consciousness and the consciousness of others is raised, that what needs healing is healed and that blessings and light should fall on the darkest corners of the universe.

I then use whatever source of water I've decided upon, whether bath or shower, or sometimes I simply ladle water over me while silently chanting that I am cleansed and whole. When that is done, I visualize a protective coat around my shining aura, close my chakras one by one leaving my root chakra open to ground me, dry myself and put on my caftan or whatever garment I choose.

Doing this even just occasionally will make you feel wonderful. But simply having a shower with conscious intent to cleanse, heal and protect will do. My children used to laugh at me when I came home after work and went upstairs saying I was going to wash the day off. But that's how it feels.

Now that's all well and good, but you might find that you need to cleanse and protect yourself very quickly. Someone may have dumped all their psychic pain on you, hurled abuse at you or whatever. Just with a thought, set your intention and imagine white light pouring all over and through you, cleansing, healing and balancing. Then close down and imagine a golden coat all around your aura to protect you.

You can also set up protection when you know things are going to be difficult by erecting a pillar of light in which you sit. Put it around someone else also if you wish. I often erect such a pillar around myself and my patient and call in angels to help as well. We'll talk of angels and helpers in Chapter 10.

Closing Down

You'll find a closing down ritual at the end of the meditation on page 58.

Three

The Heart Chakra

Infinite love is a weapon of matchless potency.
It is the summum bonum of life. It is an attribute of the brave,
in fact it is their all. It does not come within the reach
of the coward. It is no wooden or lifeless dogma but a living
and life giving force. It is the special attribute of the heart.

—GANDHI

Antoine de Saint-Exupéry, in the inspirational book *The Little Prince*, said, "It is only with the heart that we see rightly. What is essential is invisible to the eye." We now look more closely at how we "see rightly" with the heart. For it's here that we encounter the great energy of love, that grandest of feelings that enables us to extend ourselves in a way we may never have thought possible and touch the heights and depths of human emotion.

That you're lovable and greatly loved is not in question, except perhaps to yourself. That you're capable of great love—as light as a whisper and as deep as a groan—is also a certainty, though that will become more obvious as we move to later chapters. The aim is to love consciously, with full awareness and dynamic purpose, and yet to achieve this as effortlessly as breathing—by being just who we are.

Often we've been "loving" in the way "love" was demonstrated to us as children, or have decided not to love at all since the love we knew was laced with hurt, conditions and a high price. Sometimes old wounds and misunderstandings about what love is get in the way of learning to love healthily. If what we see as love is actually possessive and sick, that's all we can give. But the good thing is that human love has been learned, and it can be unlearned and relearned too. In following chapters we'll look at how we learned our particular brand of love and at how you can develop a new brand if you wish. You can choose to do it differently. You can choose to break all the rules you ever learned about how it should be. You can decide not to play the games you've played in the past.

Since we're beings gifted with a physical body, emotions and intellect as well as a soul, we'll be using all of these on our journey. Though opening our chakras and allowing love to flow can feel wonderful, if we want long-lasting change rather than a quick fix, which leads to disappointment, we need to use all of ourselves.

Every quality, emotion, talent and gift can be traced through the chakra system. The age when we suffered trauma affects its development, preventing the free flow of energy. Any problems between the ages of 12 and 16 will affect the heart chakra directly, but hurt at any age will have a domino effect, stunting the function of the rest of the energy chain. We can heal those blocks if we're willing to work at it, use our energy to access greater gifts than we ever imagined and live in a way that's directed by love.

Center of Love

Here, in this wondrous chakra, is the birthplace of human love. John O'Donohue in his sensitive *Anam Cara* talks of love awakening in your heart being like the dawn breaking—anonymity being replaced by intimacy, fear by courage and awkwardness by gracefulness, bringing us a new beginning.

Every chakra brings us love in some form. But the human heart and its capacity to love is a constant wonder. As the present rolls out, second by second, prolonging the eternal moment for ever, the heart responds with a stream, sometimes a raging river, but always an ever-present blessing of love. The heart caresses the soul, and on the wings of love we extend ourselves to bless and be blessed by others. Spending a moment whenever you think of it to send a loving thought out into the world will do amazing good and reap untold benefits for you and all of humankind.

The heart chakra, at the physical center of the body and the center of the chakra chain, is a pivotal point—a place of balance and integration at the intersection of several axes, holding them in perfect equilibrium. As it glows with emerald light, it connects the lower centers that deal with the physical world with the higher centers that deal with the spiritual. As these two energies (matter and spirit, earth and cosmos) meet and unite, the force released is love—a powerful, life-giving energy that can sustain us in times of hardship or disaster, can soothe the agitated soul, can heal the broken heart, can move mountains and can render us free, whatever the physical reality.

It also balances the relationship between the human nature and ego of the lower chakras and the increased awareness and more spiritual nature of the higher ones. It helps hold us secure when we fall in love (see Chapter 8)—those chakras below keeping us rooted when we could so easily lose our grounding, our love then having little substance to sustain it.

A healthy heart chakra allows us to expand, increasing our capacity to love without barriers, to feel unity with our fellow human beings whether we know them or not and to live in happiness. When our heart is closed, not only do we lose loving contact with others but we cut off the flow of energy within ourselves.

Love, Love, Love . . .

Let's look at love—we'll find out more about it with every relationship we view.

It is only through love that we can attain communion with God, wrote Albert Schweitzer, but actually it's only through love that we can attain communion with each other too. Love holds us together. Love, loving and being lovable are natural states. Love is active, dynamic and creative and enhances and sustains us as nothing else can. It flows from one heart to another, awakening the divine and warming and making cherished lives that may have been a cold, barren landscape. Our love communes not only with the divinity in others, but with the great divinity of which we're all part.

The heart allows us to open to our gifts, to share them generously with others while prompting us never to forget ourselves. And since to love is to want to give the best, it prompts us to be the best that we can be, to develop the talents we've been given so that we can use them to enhance the lives of others. Thus it prompts us to continue on a path of self-development and to constantly extend ourselves so that we have the best to give.

Pitirim Sorokin in his wonderful dissertation, "The power and ways of love," stated that love creates love. It's only by loving others that we can create human love in our lives, though divine love is always there in abundance (see Chapter 10). And love is magic! The more we give away, the more we have. And the more we love, the better we feel about ourselves, the happier we are, the more creative we feel. A bonus is that those who actively love, live longer!

Love is the most therapeutic commodity known, a powerful antidote to all ills, to hatred which infects great areas of the world and the fear that prevents us from denouncing it. It helps children to grow into responsible and peace-loving adults, it prompts great acts of courage, it flows across boundaries of race, creed, color and political doctrine and can eventually abolish the pain of the world. It can help those with criminal tendencies to turn back, it can heal sickness and it ennobles everything it touches.

Opening to the love for the Divine, which involves both heart and crown chakra (see Chapter 10), enhances every aspect of life and allows us to look afresh at every human being in their full human glory, going about their everyday lives often unaware of their own divinity. As the great peaceful warrior Martin Luther King, Jr. declared, "Unarmed truth and unconditional love will have the final word in reality."

Love—Eros to Agape and Beyond

The more we can clarify what we mean by love, the more we can live in balance within ourselves and the world. Chapter by chapter we'll be looking at different aspects of love, and in Chapter 10 at that deep and utter longing that calls to us from the depths of our soul and beckons us home—our love for the Divine.

Love just is! Each of us is a manifestation of love—it's what we're made of. So it's not something we have to create; merely something we must uncover and become more aware of. There are no barriers to our loving and being loved unless we've erected them because of our pain or our training.

And love is love is love—but it's like a beautiful diamond, it has many facets. It's not new to complain that the English language has only one word for love. Borrowing from other cultures can help us dissect love and study its nuances. This isn't merely academic. Bestowing on a loved human being the passion that rightly belongs to the Divine may leave them no alternative but to escape the intensity, leaving us bewildered and bereft. Being erotically intimate with someone with whom a platonic love would be more appropriate can only lead us into trouble. So let's try to examine it.

Eros was the Greek god of love. Later Freud in his psychoanalytical theory talked of eros as the life instinct, the source of all impulses that serves each individual in self-preservation and reproduction. He was talking about the love of the lower chakras, particularly the root which, as we saw, concerns itself with sex, though the sacral takes us to sexuality and sensual, erotic love. Sam Keene in his book *To Love and Be Loved*, defines eros as "the force that weaves the strands of your DNA to create a future that transcends every past, your questing consciousness, your life energy."

Agape is that gentle platonic love that exists with deep commitment though perhaps less passion and without a sexual element. It has also been said that the love with which the Divine approaches us, the paternal benevolence of God, is agape love, while we approach with a striving eros.

Philos is the benevolent love of humankind, from which the words philanthropy and philander are derived.

As you see, each of these shows a different face of love.

Ancient Greek has three other terms which help tease out some of the strands. *Himeros*—the physical desire of love; *anteros*—the answering exchange of love; and *pothos*—the spiritual aspect of love that drives us on to search for the Divine. In chakra terms, *himeros* is the love of the root and sacral, with *anteros* both at the sacral and to some extent at the heart. *Pothos* is the spiritual love of the brow and the crown.

Obviously the love that involves sexual passion is different from the love of parental instinct. And the love that holds us together as family or social group (see Chapter 9) is different again. The quality of love of the heart is different to that of the sexual, passionate love of the sacral chakra and from the power and will of the solar plexus.

The love of the human heart is a constant, enduring state of being, radiating ever outwards whether or not there is any particular object upon which that love is focused, content to simply exist. In contrast, the love of the sacral always has an object of desire.

Characteristics of Love

Several characteristics are common to that bond of love that unites us, whatever the relationship.

ACCEPTANCE

The heart chakra asks us to accept ourselves as we are and to use this as a launching pad from which we can raise ourselves to better things. Better understanding, greater courage, true forgiveness and acceptance of others with compassion for who they are, and how they came to be as they are, are possible only when we've truly accepted ourselves. Acceptance does not imply complacency, but rather a base from which to improve and grow.

COMMITMENT

In loving, there's always commitment to the welfare of the other and to the love itself, though this is different from committing to a life-long relationship.

PASSION

Passion is that energy that allows us to work beyond fatigue, to be unaware of our surroundings, to be enthused by the gods, to emit a stream of practical love, to pour ourselves into what we do. To lose our passion in its broader sense is a partial death of the soul. However, though passion is an essential part of some human love (see

Chapter 6), beware that it doesn't strangle. Hold gently or you may lose that which you desired.

CREATIVITY

Love opens our creativity in a way that little else can. Witness the great poets and composers whose works depict the opening of the heart in love or in grief for the loss of the beloved. Love is a dynamic and creative force that can enhance the lives not only of those we love but of everyone with whom we come into contact, and beyond. In truly loving, without selfishness, we're prompted to desire joy and peace for the rest of the world. Though creativity is kindled in the sacral chakra and comes to blossom in the throat, it's with the breath of love that it flowers fully.

FREEDOM

The bonds that hold us in love are flexible enough to allow movement and growth. Love encourages our freedom to become the best that we can be while urging us not to impose ourselves or our value system on others. As Antoine de Saint-Exupéry put it, "Perhaps love is the process of my leading you gently back to yourself." This is certainly so in professional loving (see Chapter 9). Love that binds with attachment strangles and encourages codependence rather than being energizing and expansive for both parties.

CHARITY

Charity is sharing what we have with love. It comes not from superiority or from a desire to be seen to do good but from a simple and loving desire to share what we have with those who for some reason have not. It's essential that we see the recipient as our worthy equal.

Charity is a means of spreading out the gifts of the universe, but more than that, it sets up a flow of energy and a stream of love throughout the world. As we donate a token of our energy, opening our hearts in the process, love flows and both the giver and the receiver are nourished in the loving transaction. Charity is a thing of joy: it is given freely, expecting nothing. Giving out of duty, from our mind rather than heart, reduces the potential of the gift in that the spiritual, nurturing element, which is much greater than the material, is missed by both. Charity, it's said, begins at home. Give to yourself first in terms of love, forgiveness, acceptance. Giving in the form of teaching—being a mentor, sharing your skills—can be more empowering than material gifts.

DETACHMENT

When developing the heart chakra there is a point at which detachment occurs. I remember it well as a sad, lost feeling as the heart bonds I had with many people began to soften and loosen and, while my love for them remained the same, I could feel a kind of floating gap develop between us. This is detachment. It's a greater development of love than attachment because of the absolute freedom it allows. It enables that part of "I love you" that says, "I want you to be the best you can be whether or not that includes me." It allows for the other to continue to grow and develop way beyond us if that is what they're capable of. It's the development that allows us to understand that wonderful quote from Kahlil Gibran in *The Prophet* when talking of children: "You may give them your love but not your thoughts, for they have their own thoughts. You may house their bodies but not their souls, for their souls dwell in the house of tomorrow, which you cannot visit, not even in your dreams. You may strive to be like them, but seek not to make them like you. For life goes not backward and tarries not with yesterday."

PARTNERSHIP

Loving often appears to be an unequal partnership—the love of a parent for a child is far beyond that which the child appears capable of in return; the love of one for another may be unrequited; professional loving asks for no return. Nevertheless, a partnership exists on a much higher level that ensures that there is freedom and empowerment for both people involved. In fact, on some level, the partnership is always one of equal benefit.

ENERGY

Each heart is stimulated by the joy of love and the sense of connectedness and appreciation of the other. The release from isolation and aloneness results in a rise in energy for both parties. The opening of the heart chakra also allows energy to flood the system. Usually there's an increase in physical energy, at least for a while, which mirrors the spiritual energy.

DISCIPLINE

Though there's a place in love for joyful abandon, the daily discipline of love strengthens our ability to remain constant among the distractions of life. In busy lives there's much to attract our attention and lead us to neglect that which we love. Being conscious of our duty to show our care for those we love enhances the quality of love.

RESPECT

We need to respect not only the desires, wishes and rights of the other, but also the fact that we're witnessing another manifestation of the Divine in action. We have no right to assume that we know better than another where they're going or what they need to do. True love also respects the right of a friend to have other friends, time for solitude and individual hobbies and interests.

CONTINUITY

In truly loving there is an air of continuity. Even when the passion of a relationship is ended, if there was true love, friendship can remain (see Chapter 7) and a desire for the well-being of the other, for their continued growth, for their happiness. In loving but leaving (see Chapter 8) we're often fulfilling that commitment to continuity even in separation, since staying together would do damage. Children in particular need continuity in the love shown to them by their parents or major caregivers.

FORGIVENESS

Lack of forgiveness is perhaps the most common block to truly loving and to moving on in life. We stay stuck, holding someone on a hook while of course, in order to do so, we must continue to hold the other end! We need to forgive, and also to accept forgiveness for ourselves. It's a pity to let someone take up part of your heart and stay fixated on something that's past. Loving means letting go, and sometimes it also means deciding that the relationship as it was is over.

GENEROSITY

Beware too much generosity! Sometimes the gifts we wish to bestow are too much for another to receive and our outpouring does little but overwhelm and offend. The loving heart sensitively holds back to allow autonomy and identity to dictate progress. Sometimes too much "loving" can be too rich a diet and can rob the recipient of the joy of self-realization. All we need to do is to be there and if necessary nudge the other person a little along the path of appropriate evolution. If ego gets in the way (see Chapter 4), our generosity is likely to try to force others into becoming clones of ourselves.

COURAGE

Courage comes from the heart and is often a response to a challenge to act with integrity even though that may be difficult. We also need courage to stay with love when the going may be tough, to work on what challenges us in relationships and to know that we're learning something we need to know. But sometimes we also need the courage to leave when we know that the situation is destructive for either party.

POWER

Though power is housed in the solar plexus chakra, the power of love is the greatest power known to us. We have the power to change ourselves, our lives and our attitude, among other things. The power of love can heal and change the planet and everything on it. Sending love is a powerful act: it can light a candle in the darkness of fear and hatred.

TOUCH

Touch—in both the sense of being touched or caressed and of being moved by beauty or sadness—is directed by love and is an essential part of loving. It has been said that a touch is worth a thousand words. Make sure, however, that touch is appropriate and welcome.

COMPASSION

Compassion is the emotion we feel for the misery and pain of others. If we're compassionate, we're affected by the joys and pleasures, upsets, sorrows and wounds of others even if we don't know them. Compassion is part of love, both human and divine. But though we may feel compassion, we also need to remain detached and take care not to rob others of their chance to learn, since it is the painful times that thrust us forward into growth.

EMPATHY

Empathy is the gift of being able to stand in the other person's shoes and see how it feels. It's not synonymous with sympathy, which tends to lead us to collude (see page 254). To love fully we need to be sensitive to the needs, desires and feelings of the other so that we do not trample and hurt them unnecessarily.

INTIMACY

Intimacy is the result of trust, openness, honesty and the willingness to be vulnerable. In intimate relationships there is sharing of power, control and nurturing, with an easy alternation of roles if necessary. Intimacy is in the way we talk and listen, laugh together, support each other, and in the quality of our loving interactions. Though erotic intimacy can be part of the relationship, it isn't necessarily so.

AFFINITY

Affinity—that attraction of one to another based on sympathy and natural ties and which manifests in warm affection—leads to bonding. The resultant connection brings new balance and stability to each person separately and also forms a new entity, the relationship, which has its own separate identity, much as the affinity of two elements results in bonding and formation of a new chemical compound. Affinity is created by unseen signals (see Chapter 8) which indicate that each has something the other needs to render him or her more whole. Sometimes affinity is based on sameness, with a sense of homecoming and peace within the bond. Whichever the mechanism, each heart chakra searches out something that enhances both the self and the other, with an increase in harmony, joy and peace for both. Affinity is an integral part of a relationship, whether of lovers or friends, and it secures the two in a cohesive whole—bound, yet free; constant yet forever changing and evolving; mutually supportive and nurturing; simultaneously teaching and learning.

Heart Recognizes Heart, Spirit Recognizes Spirit

Some of my most important lessons on love were learned while working as a visiting psychiatrist to a high security prison. The crimes committed by some of the people I worked with were dreadful, and in every case my heart went out to the victims and their families for whom forgiveness must have been difficult if not impossible. But I could eventually see what had brought the perpetrators to the point of committing the crimes. Also I could see where love earlier in their lives (not necessarily by parents, some of whom had loved greatly) could have helped avert what had become an inevitability. Though of course each was on his path.

I also learned that, though it's never too late to love and we need to keep our hearts ready to hold others in love, for some the damage is so deep that healing it in this lifetime is probably impossible. That doesn't excuse us from doing our best and loving anyway.

Loving the unlovable . . .

Sometimes love strikes us in the most unexpected ways and is so powerful that it alters our course, opens our eyes and leaves us changed forever.

Many years ago I was the psychiatrist on call one night in a hospital in the northeast of England. An elderly man was brought in, a vagrant who'd been living under one of the bridges over the River Tyne. He'd been causing a disturbance as he shouted abuse at the hallucinatory voices he perceived. He'd also been violent to those who tried to bring him to the hospital, which he perceived to be a place of prison and torture. He continued to cause a disturbance when he arrived, being aggressive towards the nurses, of whom he was afraid, and railing against the abuse of his rights.

He was filthy, infested with lice and had long hair and fingernails. The dedicated nursing staff were having a hard time, taking turns being in the room, which they often had to leave gagging.

Usually the nurses, wonderful as they are, would clean up such a patient before the doctor was called, but on this occasion they called me and warned me about what I would encounter when I entered the room. They hadn't exaggerated.

As always when attending someone disturbed, I calmed my aura and got still within myself before entering the examination room. I had my heart open to bond with him in whatever way he was capable of connecting with me, and my crown open to draw in whatever help I might need. There he sat, crouched on the examination table and the stench filled the room. My stomach heaved and I tried desperately not to show how nauseated I felt. But in that moment my eyes met his. And there followed an amazing phenomenon I didn't expect.

It happened so fast that I was only aware of an instantaneous shift in consciousness. In that split second, my spirit recognized his, and vice versa, and a bond was forged between us that included our hearts, solar plexus and crowns. He held my eyes and I his as we both visibly relaxed; my desire to vomit disappeared and I was no longer aware of the smell in the room. Silently my heart heard his call for me to approach him and he allowed me to take his hand. He also allowed me to remove his clothes, to wash and bathe him, to cut his hair and to be with him. He was beyond speech for some time. The abusive language, which had been his only defense, subsided and was replaced by silence, but I nevertheless received deep communication from him.

He was a great gift to me. I would never forget that magnetic connection on all levels with a human being I didn't know and with whom it might have been difficult to relate. That moment of recognition where my spirit recognizes yours and rejoices brings into consciousness the fact that there's no separation between us—that I'm part of you and you're part of me, and that what I do for you, I do ultimately for myself and for all the world. This is spiritual love, soul love, which is simultaneously human and divine.

He also demonstrated to me that such a powerful connection could soothe and heal without my needing to do anything more. It was a great lesson in love made the more precious because many, including himself, saw him as unlovable.

It was a great privilege and honor to be able to serve him.

Positive experiences, one of which is to be loved, no matter how briefly, last us our whole lives. The outcome isn't our business: all we can do is love and let go.

Some years after my stint at the prison, a young man I'd worked with for about three years came to my home unexpectedly while I was out. It could have been frightening that he had found my home address and sought me out. But he and my teenage daughter, a very loving soul, had a pleasant chat about his gratitude while he tried to repay me by making recommendations on how to burglar-proof my home. He'd felt the love and was giving it back in the only way he knew how.

If we can allow our hearts to open to others, no matter how annoying, debased or repulsive their behavior, we can, on some level, become a fellow traveler as they tread their path and connect with love.

Healing

Healing is a function of the heart chakra combined with an open brow chakra and a crown that allows the in-flowing of divine energy. Healing is about making whole and reinstating inner balance, peace and flow. It's a flowing of pure love that can alter physiology and chemical composition as well as soothe fevered emotion. Any discourse on the heart chakra would be incomplete if it did not mention this phenomenon.

Illness is a cry of discomfort from the soul. It tells us that all is not well. Lack of inner peace sets up vibrations within the physical that alter function and physiology. Over time, inner turmoil results in such stress that physical as well as mental changes occur, the consequences of which may be far reaching in terms of illness. Since illness comes from the soul, is taken up by the mind and presented by the body or emotions, spiritual help is essential to healing. Without this element the soul simply calls again and the body or mind is presented with a different problem. Often, however, by the time we ask for help, illness has such a hold on us that we need to accept the use of external agents such as medication or even surgical intervention as well as spiritual.

Healing brings us back to that which enables us to feel whole if illness, disability, surgery or infirmity has rendered us less than physically intact. It allows the fear of illness or even impending death to disappear.

What you're doing in reading and working through this book is self-healing. If we want to channel healing for others, we ourselves need to be as well as we can be. It's difficult for someone to feel healed if the healer is surrounded by a less-than-joyous aura.

If you choose to talk to a healer and you're aware of her ego, then be cautious. But don't mistake the exuberant joy of the healer about someone getting well as pride. That childlike response to the magic of healing may well be a sign of great humility. Also don't be afraid that you're not worthy to attempt to help heal someone because you yourself aren't feeling good. The man I mentioned on page 150 did some remarkable healing with me and taught me many things despite his own pain.

What's essential for the person who's channeling the healing is to let go of attachment to the outcome. That's not in our hands and depends on many factors, not least of which is the person's readiness and true desire to be healed. Healing will always occur, though perhaps not in the way or the time frame you expect. Make sure that you cleanse, protect and ground yourself if you're involved in healing work.

Most mothers have from time to time healed their children, if only informally, by holding and soothing when a child is ill, kissing better the grazed knee and giving words of solace, encouragement and comfort in times of distress. Often all that's necessary is the

Love bringing freedom in the face of disaster and injustice

Reading Dietrich Bonhoeffer's Letters and Papers from Prison, *I was struck by his spirituality and lack of bitterness and hatred in the face of injustice. Pitirim Sorokin talks in the introduction of* The Ways and Power of Love *of his incarceration and death sentence and yet goes on to the most remarkable dissertation on love, seeing it as the only way forward for the planet. Dr. Victor Emil Frankl talks in his autobiography of using humor with love to survive imprisonment and the threat of the firing squad. Those who've had near-death experiences are almost invariably changed, choosing to live their lives in some kind of service, with a new understanding of life and its meaning.*

All have discovered that with love we're free, no matter what's happening to our physical selves.

desire that healing should take place. Not as we might want, plan it or visualize it, but in whatever way it will benefit the higher good of the other and be in line with their own development. We can only desire what's best for this whole person now. And in some cases we must accept that it's for their higher good to have a means to let go of the physical and be free to "die."

This is why one of the features of the healing heart is to be detached and leave the other free. Sometimes, despite the grief of those left behind, there's relief that someone died. Relief that the person is now released from suffering; gladness for the life they've shared and that their loved one has now gone on.

Healing is always beneficial to both the person channeling the healing and the recipient of the healing energy. The healer cannot fail to receive healing as the energy flows nor to feel joyful at being privileged to be part of the other's healing.

There are many texts on healing—of yourself and others—and should you wish to follow this more closely, I refer you to my book, *The 7 Healing Chakras*, and *Hands of Light* by Barbara Brennan.

Fear

Our thoughts and actions are based on either love or fear. There's no other choice. If we feel no love in our hearts or around us, we often act fearfully or cover the fear with anger.

Even if we feel that there's a scarcity of human love around us, divine love is a constant reality and therefore we never need to be afraid. That's easy in theory, but less so in practice!

Fear, felt by all of us from time to time, is manufactured by our endlessly busy, remarkably powerful minds. It's real in that it troubles us, yet it is simply a manifestation of our imagination. Like pain, fear is a warning that we need to change something, to look at where we feel threatened, refuse to forgive or refuse to love. Generally, being in a state of love abolishes fear. Nothing can hurt us when we're secure in the fact that we're exactly where we should be, doing exactly what we should be doing and whatever the outcome, we're safe in the long term. That's so even if the imminent outcome includes our departure from the physical plane.

If we act with integrity and in accordance with the laws of the universe, there's no danger, whatever it may feel like on a physical level. But just as love breeds love, fear breeds fear. If you bring your-self back to a still calm place in your heart, fear can subside. Fear indicates that you're unable to trust that all will be as it's meant to be. What we focus on increases. So if you focus on the fact that you're blessed and taken care of with angels at your gate and helpers stand-ing by, your feeling of being loved and cherished will grow and you'll never need to walk in fear.

Affirmation

I open my heart to give and receive love today.
I love myself and make love flow into
every corner of the universe.

Meditation

Take yourself to your safe place and get comfortable in whatever physical position you prefer. Make sure that if you're lying down, your back is supported by a pillow under your knees. If you're sitting, place your feet on the floor with your ankles uncrossed. If you wish to be in a more traditional meditational pose, then of course that's fine.

Now focus on your breathing, filling your lungs with peace and tranquility and breathing out all the way, letting go of anxiety. Let your breathing be slow, regular and rhythmical. As you continue to breathe, let peace spread through every part of your body. Be peaceful, tranquil, all anxiety flowing out through your root chakra and the soles of your feet. Let your body and mind be at peace.

Now move your focus down to your heart chakra, in the center of your chest. See its swirling, beautiful green light, spinning and spinning. See it shining like a precious emerald. Now as you watch it spin, it starts to open, and as it does so, you see that within it there is a pink light. This is the color of love. As the heart chakra opens further, see the light start to pour forth, shining out into your whole body, filling your aura around you, bathing every part of you, filling every cell with love. Feel yourself loved and cherished; know that every part of you is beloved. Enjoy.

Now allow the loving energy to flow out through your aura and spread into the room, and with a breath, let its field spread wider and wider: out through the walls and into the surrounding area. See the love pouring out and touching everything, bathing it in pink light, healing, energizing, balancing. Let it spread now into the town where you are, and beyond to fill the whole country. With a breath, breathe it around the planet, loving, healing. Let the love from your heart touch every living thing, every point of the planet. Feel your loving connection with all things.

Now let your love spread out into the universe and send with it a thought and desire to heal what needs to be healed, to love where love is needed, to bring peace, to bring forgiveness, to heal communication. Add your own message.

Stay a while and enjoy the love pouring through and from you, healing you.

When you're ready, with a breath allow the energy to come back to the planet, back to the country, back to your town, back to your room and back to your heart. The good you have done will go on for ever. Allow the stream of love to be contained in your heart once more, knowing that you can open at will and send love and healing anywhere you choose.

Allow the swirling emerald wheel of light to close over the pink now, and slow a little. Focus on your breathing once again. Slowly and gently, start to feel your physical presence in the room. Be aware of your physical body. Move your fingers and toes. Feel yourself grounded, part of the earth. When you're ready, return to a place behind your eyes and gently open them.

Have a drink of water and, when you're ready, record whatever you wish in your journal.

Four

Being Free, Being Me

I have seen the truth. It is not as though I had invented it
with my mind. I have seen it, SEEN IT, and
the living image of it has filled my soul forever . . .
In one day, one hour, everything could be arranged
at once. The chief thing is to love.

—FYODOR DOSTOEVSKY

Our relationship with ourselves is the most important relationship there is, though one that's often neglected while we
look outside ourselves for solace and comfort, expecting others to
make us happy and complete. However, taking responsibility for ourselves, loving ourselves whatever we may do and being independent
but open to love is a mark of spiritual maturity and the only way we
come to realize our own divinity. When we've succeeded in doing so,
we're never lost for love again.

First of all, take a moment to look at what an amazing creature you are. You have a mind that has 200,000 times the capacity of
a computer and of which you usually only use about 10 percent; a
body that, if you were to take great care of it, could probably last
well over a hundred years and a soul that is ancient and connects you

to a divine source. I'm not suggesting that we become narcissists, so wrapped up in our brilliance that we lose touch with the world around us, but you have to admit, you're pretty wonderful! And you're not alone. You have around you millions of similarly amazing creatures with whom you can communicate, have fun and love, and a universe in which to live beyond anything you could possibly imagine. What gifts!

Undoubtedly, to have all this we're beloved souls. Beloved, unique, cherished. In fact we're a manifestation of the love that is the universe.

In the following chapters we'll be exploring our love and communication with various aspects of our world, but right now we're going to look at ourselves.

Who Am I?

We saw how the chakra system forms a web of energy coursing through our bodies, physical and subtle, but let's take a closer look at where we reside in that structure.

Unless we've really studied ourselves, it's rare to be able to celebrate who we truly are and to recognize the blend of qualities that makes us unique. The fact that you're different from everyone else makes you special. No *more* special than anyone else, but equally special, and your contribution to the universe is essential. It's one of the tasks of life to remember our uniqueness. No one else can give to the world exactly what you can. However small you may feel your contribution to life is, I assure you that it's profound when placed exactly where it's supposed to be. Whether that's in bringing up your children, being a brain surgeon or ploughing a field, it's essential that you find your niche and not only occupy it with grace, but celebrate it with gratitude and pride. We have a responsibility to share with others who we are, the message we came to bring and the wisdom that's ours and ours alone.

Relishing our differences is one of the joys of life and it allows us to learn from each other. Only when we lack confidence in ourselves are we threatened by the differences in others. It's then that we begin to fall into the trap of control.

Who we are today is the sum total of all the experiences that have happened to us—good and bad—in all the time up to this moment. Yes, genetics and heredity played a part, but as you'll see in the next chapter, that was no accident either. Everything you've ever thought and done, everything you've ever felt and everything that's ever happened to you, makes you who you are today. But you're more than your experiences, your body, your mind, or your soul. All of these exist together, and each is essential in making you the stunning individual you are today.

Perhaps it would help to break things down further and look at the components of who you are.

Adult Self, Parent Self, Child Self

In Freudian terms, my personality is made up of ego, super-ego and id. These have been more simply named the adult self, the parent self and the child self.

The adult self, or ego, is hopefully present in most of our transactions on a daily basis in our adult life. This part of us is responsible, practical and capable, and is generally concerned with dealing with the internal and external demands of living in the real world. Some people think of the ego as equivalent to the real self. Because the ego likes things to be organized, it's also inclined to screen what we can bring into full conscious awareness in a somewhat self-patronizing way, deciding what will be best for our self-preservation, and perhaps what's best for everyone else too. This is what prompts us to exert control over our world and sometimes those who inhabit it with us. It's the ego that jumps in with fear and prevents us from letting go enough to allow us to be fully aware of our soul. Even when we're on the brink of total surrender to spirit, the ego nags us with "what ifs" and pulls us back into our mind with doubt. Some people think that we should get rid of the ego to become spiritual. But being spiritual is about enhancing every part of us and bringing it into harmony with the rest. The ego does have its place if treated with respect. It's simply part of what makes you you.

The parent self, or super-ego, acts like an internalized parent, taking care of and controlling the child part of us that would like to run free and have a life of endless fun. The super-ego is our conscience and is concerned with our morals, with guilt and shame. It tells us what we should and should not be doing. Sometimes it scolds us and makes us feel guilty for doing something wrong, for not showing up on time, for behaving less than responsibly. In some people it's overdeveloped and can ruin things by being more like an ever-present policeperson than a loving parent.

The child self, or id, is the fun-loving, playful, childlike, mischievous and sometimes badly behaved part of us that would love to have endless fun with no responsibility and no limits. It's that part of us that likes to reduce the pain in life and enhance the pleasure. It loves to give free rein to our primitive instincts and impulses. Its desire for pleasure causes inner conflict with our ego, which sees the reality of things. It also conflicts with the super-ego, which demands responsibility and decorum. The problems caused by conflict between these three can last a lifetime unless we sort it out.

Though classification is useful to help us understand and analyze the workings of our mind, it's simply a theoretical creation and cannot conceive of the boundless wonder of the soul. And since it's a creation of the mind, in totality *we* must be far greater than anything our mind can possibly create.

To truly perceive the wonder of our divinity and the endless mysteries of life and love, we must use the soul. Sometimes as we try to do this, it feels as though we're existing on two planes simultaneously. Our soul encourages us to rise and allow the stream of neverending love to consume us. The ego pulls us back with worldly worries, with competition, needs and desires. Being asked by our soul simply to let go of the worldly and trust in the constant stream of abundance that is already there can fill us with nagging anxiety. What if it really isn't so? What if the supply dries up? What if it was merely a fantasy after all?

This is what keeps us from entering and holding onto that wonderful state where everything is not only possible—everything just *is*.

Our Bodies

If our minds are merely creations of our souls, then where do our bodies fit into the scheme of things? Our body is an energetic creation made and fueled by the things of the earth, which houses our soul and gives us form so that we can exist and function in the world. It's what makes us visible and tangible. It renders us human so that here on earth our soul can experience itself along with other souls that are currently in human form, feeling human emotion and sensation. As such, it's our temple housing our soul, though in fact, since our soul light can be seen around us (see Chapter 2), it could be said that our body is in our soul rather than the other way round. While we stay here on the planet, until it is time to return to whence we came, we have a responsibility to keep ourselves grounded and keep our vehicle—our body—in a good state of repair.

Soul and Spirit

All of us are spiritual beings, although at present in human form. My soul is an endless part of me that has lived forever, though my body may have taken on various forms. (We will discuss this again in more detail in Appendix 2.) My spirit is part of the great consciousness we call God, Allah, Jehovah, the Divine, the Higher Power, the Universe and many other names, depending upon our belief system.

My spirit connects my soul with the body of God. Though my soul is an integral part of me, always present, I need to raise my consciousness to have a connection via my spirit with God. This process, sometimes called transcending, may be achieved through prayer, meditation, chanting, music or simply by slowing my breathing a little and asking for such a connection. It becomes easier and easier to transcend the more we work on clearing a spiritual path. Transcending allows me to have experience, gain knowledge or appreciate things that are not of the human world.

Regaining Our Peace of Mind

We can use the analogy of the sea when discussing peace of mind and how we allow it to become lost. Though there may be a storm at the surface (the ever-changing emotions), the bottom of a deep sea remains calm and serene. However, where the water is shallow, the sand on the sea bed is whipped up and forms sandbanks, which can become semipermanent structures. These sandbanks are the difficulties that build up in the subconscious if we're constantly troubled by disturbed emotions or thoughts. They can cause us to have turbulent lives and find difficulty in coming back to a state of peace. Feeding our minds with things that disturb us, such as violence in films or the media, negativity and gossip, addiction and jealousy, may cause those sandbanks to build so high that we can't get round them. The water can no longer flow peacefully and currents disturb our daily lives. The anger and violence we've fed ourselves begin to erupt in our relationships and at work. We've lost the ability to achieve peace. In losing our inner peace, often we've lost the ability to love ourselves.

However, we can start to sort out those currents by addressing the problem of how we developed them: we can make changes, while cultivating new and positive aspects of our nature to counteract the damage we've caused ourselves. The two processes need to go hand in hand. Starting to see the best in others, having conversations where saying anything unkind or negative is banned, developing the ability to see things from the other's point of view, developing our ability to show love and compassion and be empathic while living by the golden rule of do as you would be done by, all help. Bit by bit, our inner landscape will change and we will both increase our self-knowledge and learn to be comfortable with devotion and peace. As long as the desire to do good doesn't become an obsession that in itself causes disturbance, peace can be achieved once more. It's in a state of acceptance and loving detachment that we are truly at peace. At such times we accept that though we must do our best, it's not our business to change others. Everyone is where they need to be, working out whatever they came to do. God is taking care of them.

Coming to Terms with Who You Really Are

Heredity and environment play a part in the development of personality. There are some who are born with a sunny temperament and manage to smile whatever happens and others who are more serious and introspective and find it difficult to take themselves or anything else less than seriously. Our season of birth also matters: there are many texts on astrology that could convince you of that if you have an open mind.

Some people are performing very much at the level of the personality, governed by the ego, while others are more in touch with their spirit. Have a look and see where you lie in that spectrum and you'll get some idea of how much work you need to do to feel happier about yourself and your world. You may also see that you flip from one to the other from time to time. That's not unusual as you start to work on yourself. Even those who have done lots of work will still slip occasionally and feel betrayed by or sorry for themselves, forgetting for awhile their connection with the Divine and their belief in the love of the universe. Some situations may leave you feeling powerless and it may take a little time to right yourself again. That's okay. This is a process. We're human beings and we're not expected to be perfect.

Characteristics of Those Performing from the Ego

They
- tend to be pessimistic, suspicious and negative, often seeing the bad rather than the good in events and sometimes in people too;
- are often rather morose and dull with a dry and cynical sense of humor, which may include teasing that is a little cruel;
- tend to be controlling and become upset and moody if challenged;
- are competitive and like to be right, don't like to be beaten and may behave childishly if they don't get their own way;
- have power struggles and get anxious and fearful that anyone else might do better or be appreciated more than them;
- are critical, irritable and impatient;
- are negative, complaining and tend to gossip;
- may have favorites with whom they take sides, sympathize and sometimes collude;

- underestimate the value of the gifts they have and find it difficult to count their blessings;
- are followed around by disaster, drama and chaos;
- feel abandoned and lonely and may crumble under stress despite having a strong and powerful facade;
- are judgmental but don't like to be judged or criticized;
- believe in punishment for others while finding it hard to take responsibility for their own actions;
- may be distrustful of others and have difficulty in accepting them as equals;
- may find it hard to deal with people from other cultures or social groups;
- often fail to achieve their potential.

All of us have some of these characteristics. Sometimes for brief periods we may be thrust into melancholy and be unable to see the big picture and get things into perspective. Happily, not too many of us are as closed as this. Most people, until they start to do self-improvement work, have a mixed picture with peak moments when their soul shines through—when a new baby's born, when they're on vacation and having all the attention of the person they love, when they sit with a loved one and watch the sunset or listen to music.

However, the person who's open to their spirit and lives on a soul level will show a very different picture and sustain it for the vast majority of time.

Characteristics of Those Living on a Soul Level

They
- are optimistic and see the good in all things, feeling grateful for what they have and believing in the wonder of the universe and everything and everyone in it;

- feel blessed and trust that whatever happens is a learning experience;
- enjoy seeing friends but also love solitude, appreciating time for themselves and rarely feeling lonely;
- feel happy generally, holding no resentment or bitterness;
- are usually bright and sunny, strong but gentle, taking pleasure in the success of others and bringing a breath of fresh air, joy and happiness to those they meet;
- are patient and open, discreet and respectful;
- often live quite simply, loving to meditate, be creative and have peace;
- love deeply but with freedom and detachment;
- are accepting of all races and walks of life and respectful of cultural differences;
- feel loved and protected;
- are eager to explore new concepts, grow and achieve their potential;
- see difficulties as challenges and catalysts for change;
- revel in the empowerment of others;
- accept responsibility for their actions and don't blame others;
- tend to be peaceful warriors on behalf of the downtrodden;
- because of their belief in karma, try to live by the golden rule (see Chapter 10).

Living in connection with your soul makes life simple and happy and takes away the fear of whatever might befall us. We'll be looking at that again in later chapters. For now, we're just looking at you.

Negativity attracts and creates more negativity. I've seen many patients who complain about the bad things that have happened to them, yet constantly berate others, complain, criticize and make negative comments, gossip and generally behave in an ugly manner. They seem to be unable to see that what they do to others is exactly what they complain about in their own lives.

Spontaneity

Spontaneity is a gift of the soul that makes us feel better about ourselves. Refreshing and light, changing the tempo or direction of our lives, it allows us to escape, for a while at least, from the restrictions and control imposed by the ego and super-ego. Our own wisdom urges us to do what is right for us at this moment despite the fact that we may have planned something different. Sometimes it points to new and unexplored avenues that will enhance our lives. Watch for synchronicities (see Chapter 10) that show you a new path, and allow yourself to follow spontaneously.

Being happy is often an active choice. I'm not implying that we should ignore the pain in our lives and act happy and smile when we want to cry. But we could take a positive stance in most situations, looking for the meaning in loss and seeing even tragedy as a challenge and something to learn from. We can look for the bright side in almost any situation and make that our focus. We can make a decision to look for the humor in everything. What we focus on will always increase, and what we ignore will eventually disappear from view.

All of us can learn to actively experience the gifts of our soul despite the fact that our mind is so busy creating its own world that it would have us believe that it's our highest authority. To bypass our mind and reach a pure soul experience may appear to require a lot of spiritual gymnastics. Whereas in fact it's as easy as simply becoming still, letting go and going within. In choosing peace and harmony in our lives we become awake and perceive the bliss of the soul.

Being Myself—Living My Life

We spend much of our time conforming, doing our duty, doing what's expected of us, whether that's being a good parent, getting the housework done in the morning, going to visit parents or working from nine to five. Routine is fine, as long as it doesn't become a strait-jacket! We're driven on by the inner voice that says we should be doing this or that and we hardly ever argue: we just get on with it. There *are* times when we do need to conform and to get on with the job at hand even though we might prefer to do something else. But every now and then it's worth stopping for a moment and asking whose voice it is in your head telling you to do things in a certain way. A parent from the past? A schoolteacher? An ex-husband? Or even a present one? Is that what you really want? Where is *your* voice in all this? What does it say?

I'm not suggesting that we become irresponsible. Nor that it's okay to ride roughshod over others' feelings or sensibilities. But *I* am in the driver's seat of *my* life and I won't give up that place for any-one or anything. We only get today once, so it's up to us to make it count. If we lose time by trying to be what others want us to be, to do what others want us to do, we often end up pleasing no one and wasting precious time when we could have been enjoying being our-selves and doing what makes us happy. And while we're trying to live the life that someone else thinks we should, we're shortchanging those who love us for who we are. We become cardboard cut-outs, doing what we're told and losing the characteristics that people found at-tractive in us.

Of course we can take counsel or listen to advice, but we need to make the final decision ourselves. Listening to our own inner wis-dom doesn't prevent us from making what appear to be bad decisions from time to time—but we learn even from things that appear to go "wrong." You know better than anyone else what's right for your life. And what's more, you, and only you, have to live with the conse-quences of your decisions. But be aware that there *are* consequences of every decision we make. If there's something you'd really like to do, listen to yourself, check in with your integrity, and if it feels okay, do it. If you listen, your inner voice will tell you exactly what's right.

So if you feel that you want to laugh and play, to run, to sit in the moonlight or stand outside in the thunder, to drive your car quite fast or mosey along real slow, then within the bounds of the law, do it! The meditation at the end of the chapter can help you.

Discretion and Judgement

Though mainly I vote for us being exactly who we are, there are times when it's more prudent to be discreet and exercise judgement about what we do or say. There's little to be gained by being so open that we offend or cause confusion. And saying afterwards, when someone's hurt, that it's not our problem, is neither kind nor helpful.

Sometimes we're privileged to be given information in confidence. That information is not ours to give and the only honorable thing to do is to keep it secret even though this may lead us to be less than open with others. If you feel you can't do that, it's best to say up front that you'd rather not know. And if you do know something you really shouldn't share, it's not kind to taunt others with the fact that you know something but won't tell.

About yourself, you have a right to choose not to show all of you if that's what you deem to be best.

My Inner World

As the nineteenth-century poet Henry Wadsworth Longfellow put it: "Glorious indeed is the world of God around us, but more glorious the world of God within us. There lies the land of song; there lies the poet's native land."

The world around us, which we experience every second, with every breath, every sound, every touch, every taste, every sight, every

Old scars

It's time now to introduce the concept of karma and reincarnation, though I know that it takes us into a realm that is contentious for some people. However, it has been said that two-thirds of the world's population now believe in reincarnation and karma. It has been referred to in ancient texts, by poets and visionaries, and to many of us it's the only thing that makes sense of what happens in the world.

I believe that God created us and all of the wonders of the universe and that we were given free choice. Our souls take up a human mantle and live out a human life, sometimes doing good and sometimes living in ways that are not only less than caring, but are harmful to others. Though our human form dies, our soul lives on to come again. The scars that we carry from other lives are sometimes those we're still struggling with now. Accepting this, and the challenge to heal, helps us be more loving of ourselves while seeing those around us in a new loving and forgiving light.

If you would like to read more about this, see Appendix 2.

smell, is extraordinary. It's our teacher and classroom. But how much more wonderful is the world inside us.

My 87-year-old mother, a very wise and loving woman, now confined to her bed or chair, was talking to me on her birthday of her memories of a lifetime. She talked of the smell in the upper bedroom of her grandparents' home in Yorkshire where, after the harvest, the apples were stored under the bed where it was cool. She smiled at the color of newborn pigs on the farm and the sound of kittens waiting to be fed. The touch of my baby skin and the smell of my neck as she nuzzled me in the first days after I was born, she could still sense. We shared the warm memory of the smell and taste of fresh-baked bread with butter melting into it, a treat for my sister and me when we came in from school on cold sharp days. They were as real for us both as if they were present now.

In fact, though my mother's physical world is now very small, all she has to do is close her eyes and there she is in a huge world of sights, smells, sounds, touches and tastes, some of which traverse the better part of a century.

Our inner world where we truly reside is timeless and beyond space. It encompasses all we have ever encountered in our outer world, as well as much that we have not experienced firsthand in this lifetime. Sadly, much of our inner world we devalue, fail to recognize at all or dismiss without thinking of the wonder of it. St. Augustine addresses this phenomenon in his *Confessions* when he talks of men going abroad to admire the wonders of the universe while failing to see the beauty within themselves.

Though I need to go on stimulating the inner me with new experience, because that's what I'm here for, there are already sufficient experiences in my lifetime, and in yours too, to provide a rich inner world that no one can ever take away. No manmade machine can give you such a diversity of experience and information in a split second.

Looking for Solace and Comfort Within

The discrepancy between what's happening on the inside and what's happening on the outside is no stranger to many of us. Dietrich Bonhoeffer in his poem "Who am I?" (in *Letters and Papers from Prison*), written during World War II, talked of this. While appearing to his warders as calm, cheerful and friendly, bearing his misfortune "equably, smilingly, proudly, like one accustomed to win," his inner world was filled with pain, restlessness and longing, anger, grief, powerlessness and humiliation, weariness and emptiness. He asks whether he is a hypocrite, or two people at once, but concludes that in his faith in God he is complete and united.

The inner world is more real than the outer world, and in the blink of an eye is just as present and vivid. The development of our inner world so that it can sustain us in times of sorrow, loss, tragedy or loneliness is an investment that we're wise to make.

My Relationship with Me

I hope the foregoing has helped you see what a fascinating being you are. By now, perhaps you are a bit more loving of yourself. Cherishing and celebrating come next!

Very simply, if I don't have a loving relationship with myself, then there's little hope that I will have one with anyone else. So taking care of me, cherishing me, celebrating who I am and doing the things I would love to do are essential not only to my own well-being, but to the well-being of any relationships I have. If I can't enjoy being with me, spending time alone with me, having fun with me, watching the sunset with me and taking long walks with me, how can I expect anyone else to want to? I do acknowledge that, for most people, many of these experiences are enhanced by sharing them, but try them alone with your soul. Breathe deeply into your heart and fill yourself with love and wonder. Appreciate who you are; if you've been feeling less than good about yourself, take yourself by the hand now and talk to yourself gently as you would to a friend. Tell yourself that you're starting on a new adventure in life right in this moment and that there are wonders to explore that you never even dreamed of. And let yourself just be . . . . You may find you are flooded with love of yourself and the universe that you hadn't expected.

There's no shortcut to having loving relationships with others. Cherishing yourself has to come first.

Now you may be one of those people who find that easy, and if so that's great. But I don't just mean going through the motions, I mean really getting to know yourself, as you've been doing since you started to read this book, and perhaps before, and allowing yourself to look into your own eyes in a mirror and tell yourself sincerely that you love yourself. Sounds corny? Too bad. It's what you need to do.

It may be a while before you can do that and mean it, but over the next few chapters you're going to learn even more about why you behave as you do, how you can change if you want to, and I want you to observe yourself with great compassion and with an open mind.

But for now let's deal with the theory.

How are you going to love someone else if you don't know what it feels like? How are you going to let them love you in return if you don't know how to receive love? If you don't feel worthy? If we're to try to love anyone else, we need to know what love feels like in all its nuances. Not just love with a partner, but love with some-one on the street who needs help, colleagues, those we don't like very much, those who are thorns in our flesh. We need to learn to recog-nize love in every transaction and to be aware that it's there even if it's in disguise. Can you really see the love in the eyes of the person who's giving you criticism? Or the person who's setting a limit you don't like? Or the policeman who stops you for speeding and perhaps saves you from an accident further down the road? You can learn to.

My loving relationship with me causes me to celebrate myself and to take responsibility for who I am and for what happens in my world. This gives me a sense of power and allows me to take joy in my successes and to look at what I could have done better with a sense of curiosity and learning rather than guilt and helplessness.

Decisions we make about our own spiritual fulfillment affect everything around us and also, indirectly, everything in the universe. If I send out a loving thought, the vibration of that love will affect all around me. My aura will be bright, shining, soft and gentle. If I

Celebrating me

Birthdays are very special. As the day on which we took on the mantle of humanity and began again an earthly life, they deserve to be marked, as we celebrate ourselves and those who love us celebrate our existence. Sadly, for some people birthdays are a nightmare of disappointment and dashed expectations. But from today, it could be different.

Some years ago I decided to have a particular ritual for my birthday, spending much of it alone so that I could acknowledge my humanity and commune with my divinity.

As a child, I came from a loving home, but one that was fairly poor. My child self has memories of material deprivation even though as an adult I live a blessed and prosperous life. I decided that part of my birthday ritual would be to give my child self a birthday budget to spend in any way she chooses. I decide on a small amount of money and I, Brenda, stand back and allow my child self the pleasure of choosing something she wants no matter how much my adult self wants to interfere.

The things she has bought include a lace handkerchief, a "pearl" necklace and earrings set that we have never worn, pretty gloves, candles, cream in a beautiful jar and other trivia. None of this has been a waste, for within the ceremony of these birthday gifts there has been a tearful joy, a true celebration of who I am and a gratitude that comes from beyond me. These gifts have a special place and are part of the celebration of myself, as I mark with gratitude my birthing into the world.

Perhaps it is a ceremony you would like to adopt.

come from a place of negativity and fear, I can create that around me too with jagged energy that impinges on everything, disturbing and infecting those who, unaware, come into my sphere. But more than that, the vibrations I put into the world go on and on forever, so consciously or unconsciously I can affect the whole world.

We're each responsible for the quality of life in which we live: individually, in our family and community and on the planet. If I light a candle in the darkness, there will be light. And if I allow anyone to extinguish that candle, it's my responsibility to light it again —a thousand times if necessary. Spreading love around me is my purpose in life.

You Are Enough— Loving Yourself No Matter What

I can only be me. It's the only way I can be comfortable, be creative, perform, relax and do my best. And being me is enough. Being you is enough too. You are the most perfect you there is, and the people around you are lucky to have you.

Some years ago, a friend and colleague of mine, a consultant psychiatrist, died suddenly. He'd been booked as the main speaker at a conference the following week and the organizers called me and asked if I would fill in. I agreed. Usually I'm a confident speaker, but on this occasion I was anxious, couldn't decide what I was going to say and spent much of the night before the conference in my hotel room feeling ill at ease and unable to sleep.

At about 5 a.m. I suddenly sat up in bed and felt relieved. I realized that I'd been trying to prepare to give the talk that my friend would have given, trying to approach the subject from his angle and trying to present what the conference organizers may have been expecting when they hired him to speak. I saw that there was no way I could do that. The only way I could give the lecture at all was to be me, to talk in the way that I do and to use my own style. Only then would the audience feel that what I was saying was real, because it would be coming from my heart and not just my mind.

I got up and got ready and, before I began my lecture, I dedicated what I would say to my friend, but I did it as me. The conference was a great success.

For me it was a success because it taught me a great lesson. I have something to offer which is unique. You do too. You have your gift for the world and it's important that you give it in your own unique style. By all means accept coaching or training, look at how you can polish and improve your delivery, but the essence of the message must remain yours. You need to love yourself enough to recognize that unique essence of you, and have the courage to share it with the world. You're not insignificant and neither is your purpose. No matter what, love and value yourself and have the courage to give your gifts. That's what you're here for.

Perfectionism

In Islamic countries, nothing is perfect. And things are made imperfect by design. It's said that because only Allah is perfect, everything manmade must have a flaw. Look at the tiles in the bathroom of your hotel in an Islamic country, or the design on your carpet, and you'll be able to find the deliberate flaw. Well, we're no different. We're not supposed to know it all, to get everything right. If we could do that, we would no longer be here. We all have needs too. Allow yourself that, and try to love yourself enough to have your needs met. But we should look at what are needs and what are wants. Sometimes we see them as synonymous. We can't always have all we want, but we deserve to have what we need.

We're all beautiful and unique, but none of us is perfect, thank God. What a pain that would be! However, have you noticed how some people either think they are, think you should be, or constantly worry because they're not?

We're spiritual beings here on the planet experiencing human life, and from our experiences we gain more knowledge. Only when we've learned all we came to learn, taught all we have to teach, given all we have to give and received all we have to receive will we achieve a state of perfection in this lifetime—and that will be the time to go. So all this striving for perfection is a bit sad. How about settling for being a great human being with flaws like everything else, including your Persian carpet? The need to be perfect does nothing but restrict us: restrict us in our creativity, in relationships, in work, in dealing with our children (whom we then also expect to be perfect) and in dealing with others who can never live up to our expectations. Look at all we're losing. Not satisfied to be ourselves, we're in constant competition with others, looking over our shoulder at what everyone else is doing and how much better or worse it is than our effort, and the moment, the experience, the wonder and the juice are lost forever.

Try to accept life and yourself as a constantly changing masterpiece with shape and color and texture that offer you a new adventure every day. Not perfect. Not complete. But developing and exciting, with every day a new brushstroke and a step towards perfection. The masterpiece is not meant to be complete until the final brushstroke has been placed upon it and the artist finally retires.

So experiment with life and don't worry about getting it wrong. You can't! Whatever you do, no matter how it turns out, you'll have learned something that you wouldn't have learned had you done it differently. Nothing is a failure. And nothing is lost.

Enjoying the "Now" and Coping with Change

There's nothing but this moment. The past has gone and cannot be changed. The past is for us to learn from. No more. And the present? It's to be lived to the full, every moment, one at a time. If I'm willing to be present, attentive and ready to learn, I can suck the juice out of every experience. Whether it feels good or bad, it always has something to teach me.

And the future? Well it isn't here yet, is it, and if I dwell on it I'll miss this moment and will never catch it again. I may think I can catch up, but I never can. Each moment I miss by worrying about the past or dreaming of the future robs me of the wonder and beauty of now. We'll discuss this more in Chapter 9.

Change is a constant. Nothing stays the same, but it can all get better. Even the experiences we don't like are teaching us valuable lessons. Certainly I haven't liked some of the changes in my life, and there've been times when I would have loved things to stay as they were. But that's not what being alive is about. In the end it's more comfortable and sensible to relax and allow change to occur with an open mind, welcoming whatever we can learn from it.

The amoeba has a lesson for us all. The amoeba is a single cell. It spends its life drifting along in the water with projections of its cytoplasm known as pseudopodia sticking out ahead of it. Pseudopodia (false feet) are wrongly named, I think. For really the amoeba holds its arms out to embrace its world. Along comes something it wants and it encloses it in its arms, makes a vacuole—a little space around it—and takes all the benefit it can from it, holding it gently within itself. And when all the benefit has gone, it just as gently continues through its world, and opens its arms again and lets the particle go free. Isn't that a lesson for life? Just imagine adopting the strategy of the amoeba and embracing all that life has to offer with love and gentleness and when it's time, simply opening your arms and letting go, moving on to embrace the new.

Your life is *your* life. Change it into what you want it to be. As we said in the last chapter—little steps, one at a time.

Some years ago I was on the point of signing a contract to take over a building and open it as a healing center. Many people had worked long and hard to secure the finance, to prepare business plans, to negotiate with the council who owned the building, and the project had become something of a local phenomenon. But literally the night before I was to attend the meeting to sign the contract, I had the strangest dream which told me in no uncertain terms that this was not the thing to do. The meaning was very clear to me, although it may have seemed rather odd and flimsy to everyone else.

First thing the next morning I called and backed out of the deal, much to everyone's dismay and annoyance. I have no doubt that there was ridicule among those with whom I shared the reason for my sudden change of heart, but it became obvious over the next few months that to have gone ahead with the project would have led to disaster for many, including myself, and that I would have given up my freedom to be all that I can be while being shackled to something that I had prayed for and wanted. Changing my path, even at that late stage, was essential. What was vital was that I had to be true to myself and to have the courage to change my mind and stand by my decision no matter how unpopular it was.

Affirmation

I celebrate the wonder of being me, my life, my love, my everything. I am a child of the universe and a gift to the world.

Meditation

Go to your safe place and get comfortable. Focus on your breathing: breathe in peace and tranquillity and let go of anything you don't need. Allow it to simply drift back out into the universe.

Continue to focus on your breathing with your eyes closed.

You are going to explore the remarkable reality of your inner world. Anything you do not wish to revisit will drift away into a place you will not visit. Just command your mind now that this will be so. Breathe and allow anything you don't want to visit to drift away now, leaving only the beautiful.

Now, as though you are opening the door to a fairy-tale land, start to explore the gifts you have stored in your wonderland. Look at the wealth of diverse knowledge you have and your capacity to recall and re-experience it at will. Without using your ears you can hear whole conversations again, or listen to church bells; without opening your eyes you can see the great art you have seen or the face of a loved one; without using your nostrils you can smell again the nostalgic smells of happy times gone by, whether yesterday or fifty years ago; without using your hands you can feel a caress or a kiss from long ago; with nothing in your mouth you can experience again the taste of homemade ice cream, chocolate cake or peppermints.

Stay a while and explore. Follow the memories, follow the sights and sounds that will lead you only to happy places. Smile an inner smile—and even an outer one—as you enjoy your excursion through your inner world.

Stay as long as you wish. When you're ready to return, give thanks then focus once more on your breathing. Start to be aware of your physical presence. Gently move your fingers and toes. Feel yourself grounded. Return now to a place behind your eyes and when you're ready, gently open them.

Stretch a little. Have a glass of water and record whatever you will in your journal before you get on with your day.

Five

Our First Template

Our birth is but a sleep and a forgetting:
The Soul that rises with us, our life's Star,
Hath had elsewhere its setting,
And cometh from afar;
Not in entire forgetfulness,
And not in utter nakedness,
But trailing clouds of glory do we come
From God, who is our home:
Heaven lies about us in our infancy!

—WILLIAM WORDSWORTH,
"ODE: INTIMATIONS OF IMMORTALITY"

The parent/child relationship is our first model, upon which all other relationships are based. In order to understand our current relationships we need to revisit, understand, forgive and heal this relationship. Thus we need to try to see it from both points of view —as the parent and the child—and to recognize this is a relationship that will be with us until either we or our parent dies. No matter how we might try to distance ourselves from our parents, they will forever be those who produced us, so the more we can understand them, the better.

Generations of ancestors and tradition, individual personality characteristics and life events, as well as a host of other factors, brought our parents to develop their style of parenting, whether good or bad. In our own turn, our behavior as parents is partly the result of that heritage. But genetics and tradition don't form the whole picture. In this chapter we'll also look at the spiritual aspect of this most wondrous of relationships, the understanding of which can transform our feelings about our parents and ourselves, heal the wounds of childhood and help us see our parents as men and women who took us into their lives and set us on our way.

As we get older, changing the emphasis from parent and child to mutually respectful adults and eventually to the younger adult parenting the parent, can be natural and smooth, or—perhaps more often—a rocky road. Putting the events of our childhood into context and taking responsibility for who we are as adults, without reliance or blame on the past, helps us traverse this potentially treacherous terrain. It's also very healing.

This is growing-up time! So let's start right at the beginning.

Why Have Children in the First Place?

This question suggests that to have children is always an active choice. And of course on one level it always is, though many parents would consider that having a child sometimes occurs more by accident than design. It's the natural order of things that the species should continue to reproduce and develop, and we're given the basic instinct to procreate as a gift of the root chakra (see page 24). In generations past, sex, whether in the context of intimate bonding of two people in love, or as the relief of a primitive urge, usually resulted in conception and birth, with seemingly little choice. In more recent years planned parenthood has been the vogue, though vast numbers of the world's population, whether on religious grounds, out of poverty or lack of awareness of choice, still feel that becoming parents is a hit-or-miss affair and that they have little say in the matter. Nothing could be further from the truth.

For most women and men, despite what they may have thought earlier in their lives, there comes a time when they desire to have a child. Many find it hard to articulate their reasons. Only occasionally are there logical objectives such as carrying on the family name or having an heir. More often there's simply an unexplained longing, whether or not conditions are ideal. Women who don't have a partner may be as strongly desirous of a child as someone in a longterm loving marriage. Gay men may have a yearning to become a father. Parents whose children are grown may long to have a baby in the home again. Some who are highly developed spiritually can feel the child hovering, waiting in the wings as it were, for its opportunity to be born. Those who are unable to have children are often beset by enormous grief, for years their lives ruled by the monthly shattered dream of parenthood.

Whatever the reasons for parenthood, these have a direct bearing upon the relationship between the parents and the child from the time of conception, and of course also on the child's ultimate development, particularly in terms of his capacity to love and to relate to others and to the world.

Let's look at what we might consider to be the ideal.

Two adults come together in love and respect and make a joint decision to crown their love by producing a child who will be part of them both. Conception is the natural result of loving sex and their journey begins with the excitement of finding that there's a pregnancy they will enjoy together. Despite physical and psychological changes, the pregnant mother will be happy and blooming with health and the expectant father will be supportive and loving, willing to rub an aching back, carry in the shopping and carry out the kitty litter, attend pre-natal classes and read the relevant books on birth and parenting. They look forward to the birth with joy and anticipation though perhaps, quite naturally, with some anxiety, and after a natural labor and delivery they are presented with a healthy child whom they will cherish, nurture and love. They will enjoy the challenge and fulfillment of successfully raising and interacting with their child from birth to adulthood, fielding all the challenges of family life with great aplomb, and finally become loving grandparents and even great-grandparents.

And for the lucky ones, both parents and children, that's the way it can be, though ups and downs are par for the course. But for many of us it's not that way, either as a child or as a parent.

If conception is an unhappy "accident" or the result of an undesired coupling; if the pregnancy is a burden, unwanted and rejected; if parenting is prompted by the need for security; if pregnancy is viewed with the dread of another mouth to feed; or if the motive is to right the wrongs of our own parents or to live vicariously through a child, then the story can be quite different. If the mother is alone, married to someone other than the father, depressed, a teenager, frightened, lost and ashamed, abandoned or abused, a wounded child herself desperate to have a child to love her, then the baby will obviously have a different beginning and ultimately the child will have a different approach to life and love.

In effect the wounds rather than the sins of the parents are visited upon their children, though it's often because of these wounds that the children have chosen their parents in the first place.

Choosing our Parents

For parents of wonderful children, the acknowledgment that our children chose us as parents can be both humbling and full of joy and awe. For those who had a particularly difficult childhood, I know that the concept is often a bitter pill to swallow. I do understand that, and I feel love and compassion for you in struggling with the anger and pain it may cause you in trying to accept it. Perhaps for the moment you could suspend your judgement, hold the concept as a possibility and allow yourself to move on. Take a few minutes if you need to, breathe deeply and come back to the moment. If you allow yourself to open to this concept, you will see how healing it is for you.

In order for the soul to experience all it intends to do in this lifetime, it needs a specific scenario as the launching pad—its context for human life. It therefore chooses certain particulars of birth that are invariable—the basic tenets of life that can never be changed.

For instance I chose in this lifetime to be born at a particular moment in a tiny village in the northeast of England as a female child to my two parents, and I am Caucasian. These things—time, place, parents, sex and race—can never be changed and make me unique. No one else shares my specific data, and even if I had had a twin, there would be a time difference in our births, no matter how small, which would still render each of us unique. Even if I choose to have a sex change, there remains the fact that I was seen to be female at birth. My parents were chosen by me as the ones who could give me exactly what I needed in this lifetime to help set the scene in order for me to do what I have to do, whether that included loving (as it did) or neglect, health or illness, patience or irritability, nurturing or abuse, presence or abandonment.

If your childhood was painful and left scars, you will have learned much more than I. Your coping skills will be more effective than any I will ever have because you learned them in order to survive. You have experienced things that have allowed your soul to become more whole.

The fact that our parents may not have appeared ideal, and modeled for us a less-than-perfect kind of parenting, was essential for our growth. If we came here needing to experience confusion, immaturity and possessiveness, then our parents showed us that. If we were to experience a life of luxury then they provided that also.

If we came to have our talents recognized, or to struggle to prove who we are, the scene was perfect for our needs. Though I can never condone bringing up children in abusive situations, some souls are here to experience dreadful things and to demonstrate for the rest of us that there is a better way. Please bear with me: I'll explain this further in Chapter 10. If you had an abusive childhood, please know that you are loved and that you are not to blame for this in any way.

Since you've chosen to read this and are therefore ready to do things differently, understand that, should you become a parent, the child who has chosen, or will choose, you is coming with desire for you as her parent to have a spiritual understanding of why she's here and the part you're to play in her life.

The soul link between a child and its parents is not accidental. As one generation builds on the last, moving ever forward, a tide of humanity reaching out into the future, the souls preparing to re-enter the human experience choose their place. As parents and children we're known to each other for many years before the pregnancy and birth, and the bond between us can be forged well in advance by tuning in to the soul waiting for you to be ready to be her parent.

Sometimes a special child, with specific needs, chooses us as a parent. This can be a hard road and a long one as we live out the ancient agreement between parent and child to mutually experience unusual and sometimes very difficult lives. Though there may be grief for lost potential, expectations that will never be fulfilled, there are also blessings other parents will never know. Many parents of children with special needs find a whole new life and meaning in sharing a deep, loving relationship with their children, rejoicing in successes that are simply on a different scale from those of others. Not only are the children special: they have chosen special parents who, though they may find the road hard, have special gifts that the child needs. Simultaneously, the parents are experiencing things that they too have added to their curriculum for this lifetime.

Pregnancy—a Time of Transformation

Let's have a look at the beginning of our earthly life.

Conception occurs as the sperm and ovum unite and a new entity is formed. From this moment, neither parent will ever be the same again, even if one or the other fails to acknowledge the wonder of the new life created. Ideally this is a time of shared happiness, though for many, sadly, it isn't.

Pregnancy is also a time of empowerment and transformation when a woman's connection with her innate creative ability is awakened. The souls of both mother and unborn child are keenly attuned and preparing for birth. Though in fact they connected in a spiritual sense long ago, it's now that most parents start to become aware of the first flutters of bonding with their unborn child.

Growing a new being in a sacred place inside our body is not only a biological process, but also a spiritual one. The quality of connection between parent and child and the prospects for their future relationship can be enhanced or damaged at this time. Mother and child are equal partners in this mystery and there's much wisdom in the mother's judgement as she listens to her body, heart and mind. However, though pregnancy is a natural state, medical intervention is sometimes essential: this should be as sensitive and discreet as possible, and the tendency for it to become a technological event should be avoided.

Birth—the Mother / Child Partnership

The spirit has progressed from pure freedom into the denser realms and finally connects with the soul of the child about to be born. With a breath of the divine, the soul becomes embodied in the baby, and the child is born. An awesome miracle! A holy moment.

Birth is a spiritual event. The sacred partnership of masculine and feminine has resulted in the creation of a new being, and the arrival of the child is a tangible part of the journey of the soul. The mother can best surrender to this magical time by being in an intimate and private, familiar environment, with those she loves and wants to be present. Her choice of venue, position and pain relief should be respected, and intervention kept to a minimum. Though for some, birth can be a messy affair, if its sanctity is revered, the practicalities become a mere stage upon which the miracle is performed.

This welcoming of the newborn demands minimum disturbance as parents and child commune with joy, their souls lovingly recognizing each other and bonding.

This is how it *can* be.

An account of a birth directed by the parents is given in the moving and intimate true story *Benjaya's Gifts*, by M'haletta and Carmella B'Hahn. The venue was a birthing pool prepared by her husband in the sanctuary in Carmella's home; the witnesses chosen were friends and family and two midwives. The spirituality of the event, the heightened awareness of the mother and the reverence with which the child is welcomed are reported in such sensitive detail that there could hardly be a better account.

Infancy

Infancy is the natural continuation of pregnancy and birth, when mother and child continue to bond and partner each other in a progressive series of physiological, psychological and spiritual events. From the moment the mother holds her newborn child, puts it to her breast and explores every inch of it, they're locked in a shared ecstatic experience, skin to skin, pleasuring each other with touch, smell, sound, vision and taste. This intimate interaction is equaled only by the lovemaking that ideally preceded the conception.

Adoption

Adoption has always interested me. I have wondered what it is like for the mother who lets go of her child, an adoptive parent who is given a child or indeed to be the child who is adopted. Fairly recently the reality was brought home to me, since in our family we now have three beautiful children who came to us by adoption. The wonder of this has opened my heart and mind even further to the process.

That women have borne these children and have been willing, on a spiritual level, to do whatever was necessary, however that may be perceived by the outside world, to enable them eventually to be "given" to parents who were longing for them, is a spiritual phenomenon that fills me with awe and gratitude. What agreement these children have with their natural mothers and fathers is not my business, and the agreement they have with their adoptive parents will be played out in due course. But that they have chosen to come and be loved and nurtured by a new family, to change our lives and bring us love, to allow people the joy of parenthood of which they would otherwise have been deprived, is magical.

Sometimes there is distress on the part of the person who has been adopted that their birth mother allowed the separation. But the spiritual transaction by all involved—the child, the natural family and the adoptive family—is astonishing. The adopted child can be seen as a spiritually evolved ambassador who took an unusual route to touch even more lives than most of us can.

What a great gift to all.

The human infant needs more love and care than the infant of any other species during the long process of developing independence and maturity. Though the dependent child may physically survive a neglectful beginning, without the love and care of an adult with whom to bond, there's often irreparable damage to the growing personality. Such damage may well be part of the curriculum for the soul on this life's journey. However, our aim as parents, individuals and society must be to strive to support and nurture our children as they learn who they are and develop a true sense of self and what it means to love and be loved.

Love is what helps the baby to thrive, and physical touch—holding and caressing—is as important, if not more so, as nourishment. Babies who are massaged grow and develop more vigorously than those who aren't. Infancy allows for the fulfillment of the shared need of mothers to mother, and babies to be mothered. New mothers may need to have their confidence bolstered in order to make this most fundamental time in the life of each of us a healing beginning. The universal rewards in terms of love and peace will be great.

If birth and infancy was not a time of peace, love and ecstasy for you either as a parent or a child, perhaps you would like to revisit that time and send love, forgiveness and healing to all those involved. Read again the section on our choices as we come into the world (page 61). The meditation at the end of the chapter may help you.

The Responsibility of Being a Parent

Of all the experiences of childhood and adolescence, family life has the most profound effect, and in particular how much time parents spend directly communicating with their children. Statistics show that the likelihood of adolescent pregnancy, violence, substance abuse and crime increase among young people when fathers are absent from their children's lives. Children whose parents have talked to them about smoking, drug and alcohol abuse are less likely to get involved in such behavior. Relationships and role models within the family not only help shape the character of the child but also have longterm effects on issues such as choice of partner, ability to succeed, self-esteem and self-confidence. Unless natural rivalries, conflicts and arguments are softened by love and affection, communication and understanding, there's a diminution in the sense of self, the strength of personality and the willingness of children to put themselves and their message out into the world.

Ideally, having made a conscious decision to be parents, we pledge that, no matter how tough the going gets, we'll be there for our children and honor the responsibilities of parenthood—to love, protect, teach and guide them and ensure their physical, emotional and spiritual well-being while the amazingly powerful being in our child's body starts to remember who she really is, and until her physical frame is strong enough to protect itself. Being chosen by our children as their guardians and guides is such an honor that we need to hold the task in high esteem—and ourselves, for having been chosen to do it.

It's from the world around that a child learns what love is. Not just as a word that can be spoken or withheld, but as a state of constant being—unconditional, supportive and boundless. And yet a love that is strong and wise enough to set limits. There's a poignant moment in the film *The Miracle Worker* (MGM/UA, 1962) about Helen Keller, when her teacher states that Helen's greatest handicap is not her deafness and blindness, but her mother's love which, out of pity and sentimentality, sets no limits on her behavior.

Parenthood is a great spiritual and psychological adventure, full of complexity, in which we're simultaneously observer, fellow traveler, student and partner, every stage different and challenging, until finally we recognize our child as an adult. Parenting also includes helping our children realize their potential, setting them on the road to becoming healthy, responsible independent adults, secure in their own sense of power and with a sense of the spiritual beings that they are. As the child develops, parents are being challenged by their own life changes and emerging spirituality. The parent/child relationship is always dynamic and complex. While trying to be good parents, we're often still dealing with our own wounded inner child who needs love, nurturing, affection, care and intimacy.

What's more, we are given neither a map nor an instruction book—though there's abundant literature on the subject, written by people like me who have made their mistakes too, and hopefully learned from them. Our main guide is what we ourselves experienced as children and observed in other families.

Every culture, religion and community has its own expectations of parenthood, and within each family there are traditions that dictate the way in which parents and children interact. An Italian father will have a totally different way of demonstrating love than a Scottish one; a Jewish mother behaves differently with her child than a Chinese mother. And African culture, which accepts the child sitting by the fire late in the evening listening to the ancient wisdom of the tribe, produces a different child than the one who has a strict bedtime and is not privy to adult conversation. Though thankfully we have moved on from the time when children were to be seen and not heard, there are still great variations in how much their communication is attentively welcomed.

Whether there is a tight nuclear family or an extended family system where relatives other than the parents share childcare, one basic fact usually underpins the whole: parents have a strong and abiding love for their children despite the ups and downs of life. Mothers protect their children as a tigress protects her cub. Astonishing feats of strength and courage in the face of threat to the safety of our children have been reported. Many parents would willingly break the law and, if necessary, die to protect them. However, this may not always have been so!

All parents make mistakes. It's part of what happens as we learn from our children and they from us. Love will generally help children

When it appears there is no parental love . . .

Though we expect that parents will love their children with fierce devotion, this does not always happen. Children have been, and still are, used for material gain, and subjected to experiences that injure and cripple them. We don't have to look far back to find a time when infanticide was almost commonplace, especially where children were deformed, illegitimate or one of a multiple birth. In some places even today children, especially girls, are left to die or are systematically killed.

It's difficult to say why things appear to have changed. The acceptance and availability of contraception, the possibility of safe abortion and demand for adoption have relieved many women of the anguish of unwanted pregnancy. I have no doubt that sometimes infanticide was performed in wretchedness and for the benefit of a child who would otherwise tax the meager resources of the whole family and still die. Sadly child abuse— physical, emotional and sexual—is still all too common. There is no room for complacency.

We need to send love to all those who are caught in a pact that involves abuse, asking that each side may be quickly released from this and find peace and forgiveness. They also deserve our gratitude for demonstrating how we need to change.

overcome our errors and give them a sense of security as they emerge from childhood dependency to the full maturity of adulthood.

As Jean-Paul Sartre said, even before we're conceived our parents have often decided who we will be. It's not easy to tread the fine line between guiding and setting limits while not interfering with the development of the psyche. The word "psyche" is related to the Greek for butterfly—a creature that undergoes metamorphosis and transformation. The great responsibility of parenthood is to stand back and watch as the butterfly emerges, holding it tenderly, tending it carefully and being vigilant that we neither damage it nor miss its unique beauty by trying to make it something other than it is.

Do As We Say or Do As We Do?
Parents as Role Models

The most powerful factor in a child's life is the family. Whether we're aware of it or not, as parents we are the prime role models for our children, a responsibility not to be taken lightly.

Teaching should be a loving sharing of ideas, a healing exchange enjoyed by both the teacher and the pupil. If there isn't joy on both sides then perhaps you need to reassess your method of teaching. Attentively listening to your child and talking calmly and quietly so that he can understand, and explaining details without being patronizing, can make a great difference in how your child behaves, how the two of you relate and how you feel about yourselves.

The most effective teaching is done by example. Being honest and living with integrity, being willing to say we're sorry and being courageous and confident as parents will encourage our children to act similarly. The kind of love we learn, and particularly how we demonstrate that love, depends greatly on the kind of parenting we receive. Affirmation in the form of smiles, praise and hugs when your child shows affection will teach him that this is the way to show love. Reproach or rejection teaches him to demonstrate his affection less, or at least in different ways.

Choosing to smoke cigarettes, to drink alcohol, to be abusive to our partner, to swear or to work too hard gives important messages about how to behave as an adult. Boys who see their mothers abused by their fathers grow up thinking that's how men behave. Girls who witness the same thing often grow up choosing abusive partners for the same reason.

Most of us would like to offer positive role models to our children. However, the rebellious nature of adolescence sometimes leads our offspring to oppose everything we've tried to model and teach. What we are seems only to help them define what they don't want to be. It can be very distressing for parents who've done their best to love, cherish and support to suffer rejection and humiliation as their children behave contrary to their teaching. This rebellion is a natural part of growing up and a phase that generally rights itself in adulthood when we revisit our roots.

The poem "Children Learn What They Live With" by Dr. Dorothy Law Nolte sums it all up. For instance, she points out that children who live with criticism learn to condemn, while those who live with encouragement learn to feel confident. Tolerance teaches patience, praise teaches appreciation and acceptance teaches love. This poem can be ordered in its entirety (see Bibliography, pages 301–302).

Are You a "Good Enough" Parent?

Being a parent isn't easy. No matter how we may have longed for our children, how good our intentions or how many books we read on the subject, we only know what it's like when we're doing it—when it's no longer theory and when the only person responsible for this new life is us. We have our own baggage, our own pain and our own insecurities and if we waited till we'd sorted them all out, it would generally be too late to think of having children! So the best we can do is educate ourselves as much as possible, keep calm, meditate, ask for guidance and pray—then roll up our sleeves and get on with it. Realistically, if we aim to be a good parent, with luck we'll turn out to be good enough.

However, even if you're stuck with boisterous children tearing around the house, or struggling with an adolescent you understand so little that you sometimes wonder if he's really yours, there are changes you can make that will render life more serene.

Rule number one is to try to come from a position of love, whatever's going on—and that includes loving yourself and looking after yourself (see Chapter 4). I know it's difficult to exude love when someone appears to be breaking every rule you tried to make, looking at you as though you couldn't possibly know what it's like to be a teenager and accusing you of being the world's worst parent, but in the long run it's the only thing that works.

If you're having a real struggle to parent your children, instead of blaming yourself, why not get some help? Learning to build bridges between ourselves and our children is a worthwhile exercise and it's never too late to start.

Mothering

Oh the responsibility of being a mother! From the moment of birth, much of our child's life experiences will be governed by those very early days. Not only that, but our feelings will often govern theirs. If we're relaxed and happy, then generally our children are too. But if we're agitated and depressed, angry and anxious, then the uneasy vibrations that we put out into the world will be absorbed by our children who behave accordingly. (This goes for fathers too!)

Often mothers who are fraught and unhappy complain about the behavior of their children—that they don't sleep well, are naughty, overactive and disobedient. Sometimes they're quite shocked when I point out that it may well be that the children's behavior is not the cause of the mother's difficulties, but the effect. We need to look at our own pain and sort it out if it's not to affect our children.

The bond between mother and child is so strong and enduring that it can often be damaging and destructive too.

Whose anger is it anyway?

I went through a particularly unhappy time when my children were in their teens and I was irritable and gave them a hard time. One day I sat down and looked at what was happening and then said to them that if I was unreasonable in that way again, they should say to me, "Mom, this isn't our anger."

The first time my son actually had the courage to do that when I was in full flow, I was so shocked that it made me stop in my tracks. Though I didn't like to be reminded of it, it did make me aware that it was I who needed to make changes in my life since my unhappiness was affecting us all.

I only wish I'd thought to say it to them sooner!

The mother/daughter bond often holds the child so closely that development towards true autonomy is restricted. Daughters learn about loving, nurturing and sustaining close relationships from their mothers. But eventually, if she is to explore her true identity, the daughter needs to separate. In the process of doing this there may be a phase, painful for them both, when the daughter sees her mother as a negative role model in order to free herself. I remember this as an acutely painful time with my daughter when, having always been close and loving, she decided that I was the root of her problems and that our relationship needed to be radically changed. Since it was a time when I was struggling with my own insecurities, the perceived rejection was exquisite in its pain. But she was right, and that unilateral declaration of independence formed a new basis for our now sustaining, close and loving bond.

While mothers and daughters may be struggling with their transition from parent and child to two loving adults, mothers and sons may be having different problems. The first woman in our sons' lives, we'll always have a special place. But in relinquishing that first place, control issues often surface that can cause problems. We've all heard of the saying that no one could be good enough for our sons (my daughter-in-law is!), but really what we mean is that no one could be as good for them as we've been. What a difficult position that puts everyone else in! And what arrogance on our part.

Mothering, though natural for many, can nevertheless be hard. I hope that acknowledgment will relieve many women of the guilt of never having felt they were the endless loving breast they think they should have been. Often our lives as women are ignored and neglected in the early years of motherhood. Suddenly becoming aware of feelings of anger and resentment toward your child usually heralds the need to stand back and take a long look at which of your own needs are unfulfilled and what you're going to do about it.

What Kind of a Mother Did You Have?

Though you may not be a mother, each of us has had a mother. You may, sadly, have been separated so early from your natural mother that you have little recollection of her. However, the majority of us have experienced mothering of some kind, and many women have adopted a mothering role even though they may not have children of their own. The mothering we have sets us on course for our life and indirectly affects all other relationships. Look at Rebecca, for instance.

The "best friend" mom . . .
Rebecca was 36. She was lonely and depressed, having once again left a relationship that had appeared to have potential, but which failed to give her what she needed. A beautiful young woman, she had been in a three-year relationship with a man, now 39, who was her social and intellectual match, with similar interests and with whom

she'd enjoyed fun, humor and a good sexual relationship. Nevertheless, she'd been the one to engineer the ending of their relationship and she was angry and confused, with inner conflict about what she should do now. She missed him and wanted to see him, but said that she'd decided it was better to get out now because there was something lacking though she couldn't quite identify what it was.

A bright, intelligent woman, Rebecca seemed to have little sense of who she really was, of what she wanted or of where she was going in life. Though she'd been fairly successful and had a good and satisfying job, she had few opinions about the world in general, her life or her options. The one thing about which she spoke with passion was her relationship with her mother.

Her parents had had a difficult marriage for as long as she could remember. She and her mother had always been very close, mutual confidantes and, she declared, her mother was her best friend. They discussed all major decisions, friendships and relationships together.

Rebecca had never differentiated from her mother and was often passive in their relationship, seeing her mother not only as her best friend, but almost as a saint. She hadn't developed her own style of womanhood independent of her mother, with whom she professed to have a strong spiritual bond. Spontaneously she said that she would die for her mother and kill anyone who hurt her.

Her basic unhappiness stemmed from the fact that she measured all other loves by the yardstick of her love of her mother, and found that everyone else fell short, whether friends, colleagues or partners. In teasing out what really happened in her relationships with men, it became obvious that usually, after a wonderful, passionate honeymoon phase, she became disillusioned when the normal struggles and arguments began as the two of them sorted out the power within the relationship in order to come to rest and settle into a normal loving life. Since such adjustments are often at their height in the third or fourth year, it was at this time that her relationships usually broke up—sometimes earlier, depending on the resilience of her partner. She would become depressed and angry, grieving for the honeymoon phase, believing that the person who had professed to love her didn't, since they didn't give her the unconditionally loving responses that her mother always did. Disillusionment would lead to accusation and the end of the relationship.

This pattern had been repeated in every relationship so far, and each time her mother had been waiting in the wings, her loving best friend, to pick up the pieces. What she failed to do, however, was to confront her daughter with the obvious—that Rebecca was the common denominator in the failure of all these relationships.

This style of "best friend" mothering can often be crippling, not only to the daughter, but to anyone who has the misfortune to fall in love with her.

An attempt to help both Rebecca and her mother see that the necessary shift was within their primary relationship was met by both with anger and a tighter drawing together of the bond that was strangling them both. Rebecca's ability to value other people in her life needed to be addressed. She'd been discarding good men, who had matched her well and who, given a chance, might have made excellent life partners. Rebecca's mother needed to build a new life and separate from her daughter. Rebecca needed to acknowledge that it wasn't her job to be her mother's best friend.

It took another relationship, another heartbreak, before Rebecca was willing to look at where the real trouble lay. New boundaries needed to be set with her mother to encourage her to find new friends to talk to and with whom to bemoan the shortcomings of Rebecca's father. Rebecca needed to deal with the guilt of "leaving her mother stranded with no one to talk to." After some counter-moves to pull Rebecca back into line as the best friend and confidante, her mother eventually had some counseling herself and began to deal with her life and her marriage difficulties in a much more constructive way. At last Rebecca was free to look more realistically at life and relationships and take responsibility for her own decisions.

Competing with one's children leads them to feel that they're never good enough and sets them up to have rivalries with others. Over-protection stunts their ability to learn from their own experience and to get up when they fall. Sometimes adults who fall apart following painful life events are those who've been so overprotected that they have few coping skills to help them deal with the normal ups and downs of life. However, there's a danger in going too far the other way, giving them little support and protection, leaving them feeling unworthy and abandoned with difficulties in nurturing themselves or others.

Cathy had a different problem . . .

The "vicariously living" mom . . .

A lonely, depressed girl in her late teens, Cathy had withdrawn from a potentially brilliant career in gymnastics and possibly a place on the Olympic team. But more than that, she'd withdrawn from life.

She'd been in training since the age of six, and had been poorly socialized, her friends being drawn only from those sharing the same grueling gymnastic world. By the time she came to see me she'd elected to be mute and was indulging in self-harm by cutting her arms as her way of communicating with the world. She made no eye contact with me. Her parents were obviously very concerned about their daughter, though her mother's main contribution to the interview was to impress upon me what a wonderful athlete Cathy had been and what a tragedy it was that she'd withdrawn from such a promising career.

For some weeks the only thing Cathy was able to offer at her sessions with me was her attendance, often standing looking out of the window with her back to me. Then one day she left a poem on my desk. In this poem was all the anguish, shame and guilt she had internalized. She would externalize her feelings by cutting herself only when she could contain no more and thought she would explode.

My heart bled for her as she revealed how she'd tried to make up for her mother's loss in having been a runner who hadn't made it to international standing. She'd shared her mother's sadness and sense of loss and had sacrificed her own young life so that her mother could live vicariously through her and have the joy of success through Cathy. She'd listened to her mother's stories of her hopes and fantasies and had been aware very early that it was her job to grasp for her mother the recognition that she'd failed to gain for herself.

When she was able to talk, we explored the fact that since childhood she'd known that she didn't really share her mother's competitive spirit, but every hint that she didn't want to pursue a gymnastic career was met with more passionate urging by her mother and more guilt on Cathy's part about letting her down. By now she had no idea who she really was or what she wanted. In the end she'd withdrawn, and incapacitated herself to escape the relentless pressure. It was a privilege to work with both Cathy and her mother, who, once aware of the problem, acknowledged that Cathy's happiness was far more important than any superficial achievement. Bit by bit they began to build a proper relationship in which Cathy, for the first time, felt valued for who she was and not what she could do.

Learning to be a mother is an ongoing process of refining and defining our love in terms of our needs and those of our children. One of the best indicators of how to do it or not to do it is to look at our relationship with our own mother. If we're lucky we'll have "good enough" mothering where we realize that our mother is not perfect and that we don't have to be either. Where we learn to cope by being exposed to the normal undulations of life and learn to roll with the punches. Becoming a self-assured, self-confident adult, competent but not perfect, self-assertive and neither submissive nor aggressive, partly depends on temperament, but relies a great deal on our spiritual development, which to a great extent was in the hands of our parents.

Fathering

Expectations of fathers have changed so much in the last 50 years that many men struggle with the fact that what was modeled for them by their fathers and often appeared to be "good enough" is no longer acceptable to their partners, their children or society. This leaves many men trying to parent with even less of a map than the mother of their children.

If I look at the four generations of men in my life I can see clearly how things have changed. My paternal grandfather worked, provided, was obeyed and held in respect that bordered on fear. My father was the breadwinner who supported us and loved us but was in many ways remote. There was no affection from him except on our birthdays and Christmas morning, when he would kiss us. But his love for my mother was always so evident to me that I felt included in it and nurtured by it. Not surprisingly, I chose a husband who was somewhat introverted and remote, a good man whose love for me was never in question—rather like that of my father for my mother. His style of fathering was more open than that of my father, but along similar lines, though, like my father, he mellowed with time and has finally become a very loving, active and attentive parent. Watching my son being a father is a totally different story: he gladdens my heart as he demonstrates the more open and equal style of being loving, playful and affectionate, leaving my grandson with no doubt that he is cherished.

Our first model of manhood, whether as sons or daughters, is our father, so he holds the responsibility of setting the scene for future expectations, behavior, choices and relationships. Some daughters want to marry someone just like Dad, and do. Some want to marry someone entirely the opposite, but still choose someone like their father, while others choose someone very different. Sons either emulate their fathers and become younger versions of them, even though they may have vowed that they would not, or become as different as they possibly can. Whatever is modeled by either parent is usually a lifelong legacy and though sometimes it takes a while to tease out the pattern, it's almost invariably there.

The "best dad in the world" . . .

Elaine was an unhappy woman with discontented young adult children who were fed up with her helplessness, her hopelessness and her constant complaints of illness, weakness and being unable to cope. They'd been aware of her martyr-like manipulation since childhood and none of them would buy it any more. They were angry and impatient, sympathetic with their father and losing more contact with their mother with every episode of pathetic behavior. Having established that there were no organic reasons for her exhaustion and weakness, we set off to explore her background.

Her daddy, as she still referred to him, had been a wonderful man. He'd been all things to everyone—capable, strong, a good provider and always there. He'd protected his family and controlled everything, including his daughter's choice of friends and marital partner. This fierce overprotection had not only thwarted Elaine's emotional growth, but rendered her helpless and anxious, looking constantly to others to protect her, feeling that life was frightening and too much for her to cope with. Never having matured as a woman and feeling much the little girl she'd always been, she expected parenting and protection from her husband and also to some extent from her children. Luckily, her father had chosen for her mate a strong, bright, capable man who had looked after his children well, but who now wanted a wife who was an equal partner rather than another child.

Though it was a painful journey for her as the emotional props were kept at bay while much loving encouragement was given to her, Elaine did eventually manage to grow up, finding within herself skills and talents that had remained dormant till her early forties.

Left to her own devices, Elaine would have been just as likely to have chosen a bully as her husband—someone who would tell her what to do, where to go and give her a set of rules to live by.

Those who have had perfect, "best dad in the world" fathers are set up rather like Rebecca with her "best friend" mom to have difficulties finding a mate who can measure up. But should she do so, she might well turn out to be submissive and subservient, with a blind devotion to her partner. Often, however, a marriage with a "good enough" man is marred by constant comparison to the wife's father, her husband always being second best.

Fathers who rule like tyrants are also likely to produce children who either choose similar partners, become subservient—henpecked husbands or downtrodden wives—modeling submissive behavior to their children, or become bullies themselves with little chance of equal, loving partnerships. Some such partners abdicate the responsibility of being a parent in case they should follow in their father's footsteps.

The "tyrant" father . . .

Vincent and Rachel were at the point of separation when they came to see me. Rachel complained that Vincent refused to take any responsibility for parenting their three children, rarely playing with them or being alone with them and generally giving little input to their upbringing. Peter, their 11-year-old, was having behavioral problems at school, while at home he was difficult for Rachel to manage, but idolized Vincent despite the meager contact between them. This added fuel to Rachel's fire as she desperately tried to juggle looking after the home, her full-time job and being a wife and mother. She was angry with Peter and jealous of his devotion to Vincent despite the fact that she was the one left with the bulk of the childcare. She admitted that she'd become irritable and hostile towards Vincent, and though she loved him, she felt that it would be better to part for a while rather than continue to wreck each other's lives by incessant arguments.

From their personal histories it was evident that Vincent came from a home where his father, a strict man who ruled his wife and sons with no discussion and no argument, had often resorted to threats and sometimes to actual violence. Afraid that he might inflict similar pain on his own family, Vincent had overcompensated and withdrawn from being an active parent, taking a passive role as a husband also. He needed to learn to let go of his pain from the past, forgive his father and establish himself as the father to his own children and a supportive husband to Rachel.

Those who have been restricted in their own upbringing and have been robbed of their spontaneity often become rigid parents them-selves, unable to meet their children on common ground and be flex-ible enough to accommodate differences of opinion.

Repeating the pattern . . .

This was Thomas's problem in his relationship with his 15-year-old son with whom he was in constant conflict, locked in a power struggle in which there could be no victor. Though it was his intention to broaden his son's view of the world, to encourage him to formulate his own opinions and develop good values in order to become an independent, autonomous individual, Thomas's own experience and damage often made this impossible. Only when he was willing to look at his own adolescence and see that he was replaying aspects of his relationship with his domineering father was he able to back down and allow his son the freedom to develop his own ethics, integrity and standards of behavior. He'd forgotten how much he'd resented not being allowed to wear fashionable clothes or have his hair at a fashionable length and was taken aback when I asked what was so important anyway? What could possibly be important enough to stop him from seeing his son's good qualities? His great sadness was that he thought his father had never seen his.

Just like mothering, fathering isn't always easy. Dealing with one's own personality problems, life issues and wounded inner child often takes as much energy as can be mustered. And then there's the problem of being a father when really you're still a boy yourself. Roger McGough's poignant poem, "The Railings" (in *Defying Gravity*), demonstrates the confusion suffered by some men trying to come to terms with their ambivalence about fatherhood.

Like mothers, most fathers are just "good enough"—not perfect, making mistakes, being human, but lovingly demonstrating care, protection, strength and reliability.

Parenting Pitfalls

I fell into several of these pitfalls in bringing up my own children and for that I am heartily sorry. Oh that we could go back and do it differently! If you're a parent, you may recognize yourself here, or you may see yourself as a child who suffered—or perhaps both. Don't be hard on yourself or anyone else, but see that some of these games have been handed down for centuries like family heirlooms. Every one of them can be righted, and often the first major step is to recognize them and refuse to be party to them any longer.

PUNISHMENT, ACCOUNTABILITY AND BLAME

Punishment is a concept totally opposed to promoting learning and growth: instead it only makes things worse. There's always a way to protect the truth without attacking the other's position and making accusations. This is so in dealing with our children as well as in dealing with others. After all, it's how we ourselves would prefer to be dealt with. The golden rule, "Do as you would be done by" (see Chapter 10) also holds true for transactions with our children. Would we really like to be physically and mentally attacked for what we failed to achieve or did in a manner that others don't approve of? Would it be okay for us to be shut in a room alone not understanding what it was that we did wrong? Or would we prefer to have someone explain to us, without judgement, how we might have done it differently and help us see a better way of doing things?

If we accept the principle of punishment for our children, we're more likely to accept it on a world scale. Look at the tragic consequences. Some still condone the death penalty and war is still waged. The concept is the same; only the scale is different. If we can teach our children a better way of dealing with errors of judgement, then eventually there can be peace—both within our homes and globally. Refusing to attack reduces defensiveness and counterattack. We have no right to sit in judgement or to seek vengeance. Punishment assumes that we do have that right and that we have the monopoly on knowing what's correct.

Punishment always indicates that there's blame. But blame is a facile concept. Sadly, however, the infrastructure of many individuals and whole family systems is built upon it. If someone is the scapegoat everyone else can breathe freely. Whereas in fact, we all share in the responsibility when things appear to go wrong. And we can choose to sit back, blame others and feel self-righteous, or we can look at the lesson there is to be learned. If you can see everything as simultaneous teaching and learning, giving and receiving, there can be gratitude in every situation. Life is so much easier if we can keep bringing ourselves back to the question "What am I to learn from this?" And if I'm learning something, then someone's been my teacher and I can feel gratitude, not blame. Only in appreciating the gifts you're receiving and by showing gratitude can you really love unconditionally. Our children are perhaps our greatest teachers. Therefore punishment for what they teach us is both inappropriate and misplaced and reduces their spontaneity. They do need to be taught responsibility and accountability, but punishment has no place in that kind of learning.

LABELING

Beware of labels—even if they're meant to be good ones, they're dangerous! Labeling our children in terms of what they can or can't do, what they look like or how they behave can set up lifelong self-fulfilling prophecies. It leads to expectations, or lack of them, and it may be a long time before anyone re-evaluates the situation.

I have a friend who is stunningly beautiful and very intelligent too. But as a child she was always seen as the pretty one and somehow less was expected of her in other areas. It took some time for her to get rid of that label and be accepted as bright and ambitious and with solid opinions that have a right to be heard. Labels do nothing but categorize and distance, putting a human being in a box, encouraging us to think that we know what's inside without even opening the lid.

Just imagine what happens when a child is labeled as being slow. Not only does the label stick with the child, who then perceives himself as slow, but the emotions of those dealing with this child are to some extent preset. Pity or frustration may prevent an open-minded approach that allows the genius in the child to be seen, or may stop him from being heard as a worthy equal rather than someone for whom allowances have to be made. There are too many extraordinary things your child has to teach you and share with the world to stick a label on him. (That goes for labeling anyone else, including yourself!)

BEING BEST FRIENDS

Rebecca's story on page 101 demonstrates this pitfall. It does occur sometimes with fathers and sons too. Many young boys have been introduced too early to alcohol and violent or sexual videos because their fathers want to be best buddies with them and therefore fail to keep suitable boundaries. Recognizing our unique and honorable position as parent—the only mother or father they will ever have—can help us move into a more appropriate position and let them have other people who can be their best friends.

CONFIDANTES

It may seem that you have no one but one of your children to talk to about your problems, but it doesn't have to be that way. There's always someone you can find who is more appropriate, and who will have a more objective view than your child anyway. It's unfair and abusive to give your children information they cannot process, to poison their minds about their other parent, to expect them to shoulder adult burdens that you yourself can't handle. Please find a professional or a friend with whom you can work through whatever you need to talk about. And if you've suffered this as a child (even an adult child), or are continuing to do so, perhaps you could drum up the courage to say to your parent that you no longer want to be party to hearing their problems and excuse yourself while forgiving them for having used you like this in the past. The best help you can give is to close off this route, which can never lead to them getting really well, and guide them in the direction of professional help. You may be the easiest person for your parent to talk to, and you may love the extra closeness it appears to bring to your relationship, making you feel special and different—but that doesn't mean it's good for either of you.

LIVING VICARIOUSLY THROUGH OUR CHILDREN

Though we all want our children to do well, to have what they want, to achieve, we need to be aware that what *they* want may be different to what *we* want for them. Many people find themselves in positions in life that aren't suited to them and feel unhappy and unfulfilled partly because they've done what was expected of them to please their parents. If you fit your children into a mold of your design you may miss many of the surprises of which you cannot possibly be aware unless you give them the freedom to be who they are rather than who you want them to be. And if you feel that has happened to you, stop and take a good look at your life and see if the rules and desires you live by are really your own. It's never too late to make changes—though think well and take small steps unless your intuition tells you that more radical life surgery is the way forward. How about talking it through with someone you trust (probably not the parent you've been trying to please) before you make a decision?

FAVORITISM

All children are different. Some are like us and we may feel a close and special bond with them. Or you may find yourself preferring to be with a daughter rather than a son because you can chat to her more easily. Whatever the reason, our feelings may lead us to show favoritism towards one of our children. Be careful! This often leads to collusion with him or her at the expense of other children. Confiding in your favorite sets the stage for an abusive situation not only for other children, but for the favorite too: subjecting them to different standards and limits leads them to be ostracized by their siblings and peers and may cause behavioral problems.

INTIMACY BUFFERS AND INTIMACY VACUUMS

If there's a problem with intimacy in your marriage or with your partner, then it's up to you to sort it out rather than using one (or more) of your children to alleviate the pressure. Sometimes children are used almost as human shields to ward off situations that might lead to having to be honest about one's feelings. If intimacy (not of a sexual nature, but the giving of comfort, solace and companionship, which ideally should be given by a partner) is a problem, it needs to be gently confronted rather than avoided. There are potential lifelong consequences for a child who is used in this way, as the resultant enmeshment with the parent prevents him from being free to develop his own needs for intimacy and to search out appropriate partners to fulfill those needs (see Chapter 8).

LOADING THE GUN . . .

Often one parent, say the father, is accused of being the bully, being rough and outspoken or being the "bad guy" in general while the other parent is seen as sweetness and light. But often the "bad guy" is only acting upon facts that have been fed to him by the other. In such cases the "nice" parent, in this case the mother, feeds the other with information that requires action and then backs off, leaving her partner to deal with the problem. The "good guy" manufactures the bullets and loads the gun so that her partner fires it and does the dirty work. The end result is that one parent becomes more and more peripheral while the other is worshiped and pitied for having such a dreadful partner. Not only is this an abdication of responsibility, but it's dishonest, weak, manipulative and downright cowardly. Do have the courage to deal with things honestly rather than teaching your children to sneak around telling tales and getting someone else to speak for them.

COLLUSION

Empathizing with our children is commendable and desirable, but sympathizing with them (or anyone else for that matter) often leads us to the next step of collusion. We find ourselves making allowances, having different expectations and eventually getting into a dishonest transaction where both of us know that we're not being truthful, but we avoid and ignore that fact and carry on with the fantasy we've created. Gary heard his mother tell his teacher that his homework wasn't done because he was unwell. Both he and his mother knew this was a lie. In her protection of him at any cost, his mother is teaching Gary to lie and also proving that she herself is untrustworthy. Neither can trust the other any more because deep down you both know neither of you is honest. This sows the seeds of dishonest and manipulative transactions in other areas. Having the courage to gently confront issues as they are, models to your child a loving but honest way of being that will lead them to be self-confident, self-respecting adults who live in accordance with their integrity.

DEPENDENCY

Though we usually see our children as dependent upon us, often it's the parent who's the dependent one. Sometimes we've a hidden agenda in having children—we want someone to love us, to take care of us (see page 87). But this leads to confusion about the roles within the family and to inconsistencies when the parent suddenly wants to take charge again. By then parental authority is undermined and no one knows where the control lies. If you have dependency issues, it's time to sort them out. Remember what you're modeling to your children. And if you have a dependent parent, unless you're at the age when we naturally switch roles and start to parent our parents, then you need to look to your own needs and move out of an unhealthy and potentially crippling situation.

OVERPROTECTION/CODDLING

Overprotection always arises where parents have their own issues of fear. They project these onto their children, instilling in them anxiety, feelings of fragility and helplessness and preventing them from developing the coping skills needed to get on with life and ride the waves. Unless children are allowed to fall they'll never learn to get up by themselves. Unless they make their own mistakes, they're unprepared for life. Take courage and stand back. Hold your breath if you must, but let them stumble and recover. This goes for rescuing them from difficulties into which they get themselves. Too often I see people who've never learned the value of money because their parents always paid their debts. Or others who don't tell the truth because their parents have always lied for them to authority, protecting them from discipline at school, from brushes with the law and from standing their corner in petty disagreements. This brand of "loving" is actually harmful, and one wonders whose pain such parents are trying to avoid—their children's or their own. It's usually the latter. Children need to learn that we're living in the real world. Things aren't always as we want them to be and we just have to learn to deal with it and look for the gift wherever we find ourselves. Parental patience

---

When parents have their own pain . . .

If anger or rage has become a frequent mode of communication with your child, or if you frequently overreact, look for some unresolved pain in your own past.

Janet was constantly enraged by six-year-old Tom's behavior, demanding standards that were impossible for him to achieve, criticizing and lashing out, usually verbally but sometimes physically. Though she hated her own behavior and was worried about the long-term effects on Tom, she seemed unable to stop, her guilt and shame adding to her unhappiness. She was able to recognize that something, though she didn't know what, in Tom's behavior was touching some deep and painful issue in herself. He'd become a scapegoat for all her frustration, anger and pain at never having felt loved by her father. She demanded attention and fathering from her husband and to some extent from Tom, asking him if he loved her, wanting affection from him sometimes in front of his friends. She was only partly aware of the seriously abusive, incestuous nature of her "love" and needed considerable help to mature and develop a more appropriate parenting style while sorting out her own issues.

---

varies depending upon emotional state and level of stress, and children must learn to cope with this. Frustrating our children by not giving them all that they want is actually helping them with these coping skills.

LACKING TRUST AND BELIEF

Children learn to have self-confidence mainly because of our belief in them. The converse is also true. The more we fuss, the more we give the subconscious message that they're not capable. In the long term they'll come to believe this and be unwilling to speak for themselves, lacking belief that they have something to offer to the world. Trusting in your child's competence allows her to trust in herself. Not only this but it allows her to feel free, to think, to formulate opinion, to become all that she can be. If you start to see your child as she truly is—that powerful spirit who will go into the future in a way that you cannot—you may open up to the fact that this being has much to teach you! Our children are carrying forth the human race on a new wave, leaving us behind them. We're merely the support upon which hopefully they can rely while they prepare themselves for that task. When we get that in perspective, we see our children in a totally new light. We are interdependent. Our responsibility is to hold them as high as we can to help them on their way and not to encumber them with our own desires. Nor are we to push them ahead, for we don't know their schedule, and we're not privy to who they truly are. Though on a spiritual level we're usually old friends who love each other, we've forgotten that and are simply being human. All we can do is support, help and allow them to develop into who they are while we stand and watch in wonder.

Boys Will Be Boys, Girls Will Be Girls

There's no substitute for verbal communication, but often children are not capable of articulating their feelings and instead show us what's going on: they act their feeling out (or *in*). Some adults are still having the same problem! In adolescence, boys and girls react and communicate their difficulties differently—or sometimes choose not to communicate them at all.

Boys often act out their problems by becoming delinquent, unruly, loud and rude, with fighting, drinking and drug taking. Girls may be perceived as less disturbed, their difficulties being missed or ig-

Hugs

I love—actively, professionally love—all of the people who come to see me, and at some time we get to be able to frame our sessions by a hug in greeting and in goodbye. One patient at the beginning of her session commented that one of the nicest things about my hugs is that I never let go first.

A few weeks later I noticed that Oprah Winfrey and one of her guests were talking about small changes in behavior that lead to massive changes in our lives. A letter was read by a woman who said that she had made the decision never to let go first when hugging her children. Quite surprising things had happened. Not only had the hugs been much longer than she had ever imagined they would be naturally, but they also became much more frequent and all of the relationships in the household improved.

Would you like to try that?

nored, since they are more likely to "act in." While boys hurl anger and blame at the world, girls may harbor self-blame and self-punishment. And while boys move in gangs, girls are more likely to be in cliques, though the peer pressure applies to both. Only the deviants (in the true sense of the word—those who are different vary from the norm) have the courage to be different and in doing so can be at the mercy of the rest.

Being adolescent and being different can be painful and those who manage to live out their differences demonstrate strength and courage that we would be wise to acknowledge and praise. Parents in the meantime are balancing the tightrope between protection, setting limits and letting go. Giving a little and gaining a little, they hold the reins gently but firmly while praying!

Looking through the Eyes of a Child

Children bring gifts of love, innocence, simplicity and joy. They're our greatest teachers. They come as we did to experience what their spirit chooses in this lifetime. However, as eternal, spiritual beings, trapped once again in human bodies, they're also coping with the pain of learning to be restricted. There are human lessons too.

They need to explore the world through play, using all of the environment as a teacher and their gifts of spirit and personality to learn to be responsible people and to follow a code of conduct that lies within their own integrity as they start to remember who they are and finally recognize their own divinity.

It's not the responsibility of a child to parent its parents, to be confidante, to be a marriage counselor or an intimacy buffer.

Children initially communicate from a stance of innocence. (The rest they learn from us!) And innocence is a state of wisdom: it can't perceive evil. If we try to see whatever children do from their unspoiled viewpoint we'll learn much. Though we may see ourselves as more experienced and knowledgeable, as the superior to be respected and obeyed, our viewpoint is contaminated by years of turmoil and false messages, and by our ability to manipulate. Our capacity to perceive things as they really are is often shadowed by doubt and disappointment, disillusionment, fear and cynicism. Through the eyes of our children we can learn to see the world again as it really is. Rather than trying to make your children see the world through your eyes, why not try to see the gentle wisdom and uncomplicated beauty of the world as seen by your child?

Forgiving the Past

The past is past and we're left with the results of all that has happened to us. If your childhood was sad and lonely, abusive or neg-

Seeing our parents as people

I remember a very special moment when, as an adult, I first looked at my father as a man rather than a parent. For the first time I saw the adult who had been a little boy in a family of 14 children and what it must have been like. How it was for him as an adolescent, what might have been his dreams and his desires and how many of these were lost when he had to leave his family to become a soldier. What it must have been like for him falling in love with my mother and how their lives had developed as a couple and been shattered when he received serious head injuries during the war.

From the moment I first saw my father as a man, I would sometimes stand back and look at both of my parents as people rather than my mom and dad and observe how they reacted to each other, what they said, how they showed their love for each other. I saw how they often missed the point and became irritated with each other and I saw how simple it might have been to do it differently. But most of all I came to understand how and why they reacted as they did because I understood their pains, joys and sorrows as two people who came together, had two children and did their best as parents.

Spend a moment looking at your parents as people. Think about all the problems and pitfalls they have faced and understand how hard it must have been to be a "good parent." You may feel a wave of understanding that gives way to love and compassion in a way you haven't felt before. Try seeing them as children, then take them into your heart and cherish them whatever they did, however wrong they got it from time to time.

lectful, there must be a whole host of conflicting feelings that you've either dealt with, or with which you still struggle. For whatever reason, it was as it was, and we now need to forgive the past and move on.

If you're lucky enough to have had a good solid childhood with days of laughter and sunny skies, then be thankful and send a loving thought to the people who helped shape it for you.

Perhaps you are starting to see that you made choices even before you came here and that you and your parents were in a way equal partners shaping each others' lives. If you were separated from your parents for any reason, there is still a soul connection between you, and there always will be. You can still send them love if you wish, or healing, or simply light.

The meditation that follows will, I hope, help heal the past, though if you would like to read more about this, then *The 7 Healing Chakras* will help you.

Affirmation

I send love and light to my child self and healing to the time and events of my childhood. All that I came to learn from that time I now absorb and release the need to carry my childhood with me. I release it with love and gratitude.

Meditation

Now . . .

Go to your safe place and get comfortable, focusing on your breathing as you have done in previous meditations. Breathe in peace and tranquility and let go of tension, anxiety, anger or pain. Breathe consciously, slowly. Breathe in light to heal, comfort and sustain you. Know that you are protected and that nothing can harm you. Breathe gently and slowly, allow yourself to be held in the light in peace.

Now, allow yourself to float back in time, back and back to before the time of your birth. You will not feel any of the events of your childhood: float past them and back to that time. Go back further till you are at a time long before

If your childhood was painful . . . or if you have anger or rage towards your parents, just do as much as you can of the following meditation and repeat it as often as you like. If at any time you feel overwhelmed, bring your focus back to your breathing and get grounded before you return to the room. It might be a good idea to have someone with you if you're approaching this with some trepidation. Take your time. Nothing can harm you now. Just know that you are safe and protected and that you don't have to do this until you're completely ready. You're in charge here and you're the most important person doing this work. Feel yourself loved and held before you begin.

your conception. Be aware of yourself as a powerful free spirit, unrestricted by a human body, free, free. And from this place allow yourself to observe.

See the girl who was to become your mother. From a distance watch her and see who she really is and how she is coping with becoming a young woman. Try to see why you chose her to be your mother. Stay a while observing her until you feel you know her as a human being rather than your mother. Allow her to remain in your consciousness but move your focus now to the boy who was to become your father. Observe him also. Try to get to know him as you watch him start to develop into the young man who would meet your mother. Observe them both with compassion. Take your time and stay as long as you wish, gently observing with love in your heart and compassion for these two people.

Then gently move forward in time to beyond your conception and to the moments before your birth . . .

See yourself preparing to experience new things, to grow and learn. Know that as a powerful being you had all the resources necessary to deal with whatever life has sent you. You are preparing to enter your human body. Your physical birth was not the beginning but a continuing of who you are. Gently now . . . allow yourself to witness your birth, without any pain but with joy and wonder . . . Observe the events of your birth without feeling any pain, simply watching as the stage was set for your human life. Whatever the circumstances, they were exactly right for you to start on your earthly journey, to give you all you needed to begin . . . Feel now a flood of love and compassion for your mother . . . and your father who brought you into the world to continue . . . Breathe love and peace into that time and into the people of that time. Feel the love with which you were held, both human and divine, feel the connection that has held you forever. See that the parents you chose were those who could fulfill the tasks you set for them to help you on your journey of this lifetime. See their struggle, know that whatever happened they did their best and fulfilled your needs for your journey. Allow yourself to rise above any pain. Breathe peace and love into the events and people of that time. Open your heart to shine a beam of pink loving light around and through yourself and your parents . . . Whatever needs to be healed, let it be so now . . . All that you have felt about your birth and infancy can be healed with a breath.

Take your time, then from your position as observer allow yourself to watch your infancy and childhood . . . Rise above any pain . . . nothing can hurt you now . . . Observe only with compassion, love and detachment . . . See how everyone played their part . . . allow the relationships between yourself and your parents to be healed . . . Breathe love into the relationships and then gently let them go . . .

If there is anything you wish to say to your parents now, do so and then gently allow any reply simply to float into your mind. Let there be peace . . . Let there be understanding . . . let there be love . . .

Breathe . . . Breathe light and love into you and through you . . . let it shed a glow all around you . . . feel its warmth and its healing power . . . know that you are whole . . . .

When you're ready, allow your parents to fade from your view and concentrate on yourself . . . see yourself again as the powerful being who came to reside in the body of the child . . . know your strength . . . know your power . . . know that you have all you need and more . . . know that you are exactly where you need to be to achieve all you came to achieve . . . feel yourself healing . . . Be ready to move on.

Gently, when you're ready, start to come back to your physical body . . . Breathe deeply . . . let your heart close to a point that is comfortable and one by one close your chakras (see page xxx for closing down procedure), leaving your root open to connect you to the earth . . . Feel your fingers and your toes . . . come back to a place behind your eyes and when you're ready, open your eyes.

Stretch a little. Have a drink of water. When you're ready, record whatever you wish in your journal.

Six

Brotherhood and Sisterhood

Forgiveness takes away what stands between your brother and yourself. It is the wish that you be joined with him and not apart.

—FRANCES VAUGHAN AND ROGER WALSH,
ACCEPT THIS GIFT

"Brotherhood and sisterhood" embraces those of us who are bound by blood, tradition, custom and calling and, in its broader sense, all of us who share a human existence. In this chapter I want to look at the relationships with our birth siblings. In the next chapter we'll explore friendship, which in many ways can be seen as a chosen brotherhood and sisterhood: often it holds us more tenderly and closely than blood ties ever could.

Relationships with brothers and sisters are source relationships —that is, relationships into which we were born—and are as important as those with parents for molding our personality, predicting how we'll react to friends, colleagues, those in authority and even who we choose to marry. Siblings are our first partners in many ways—in playing games, learning to cope with parents, dealing with outside influences—so they're a school for intimacy and cooperation. Sibling relationships can be tender and filled with love, closeness and beauty, a source of delight, joy and comfort throughout our lives. But sometimes it isn't that way.

Painful relationships resulting from distorted family dynamics can lead to bewildering conflicts with others and affect our ability to perform well in the world. Jealousies and rivalries that began with our brothers and sisters are uncomfortable companions, infecting our lives for years until we come to understand them, heal them and let them go. Sometimes it appears that we choose friends who are nothing like our brothers and sisters, but often somewhere down the line we find that there's a similarity that drew us together and now gets in the way.

Sorting out why we feel as we do towards our brothers and sisters is a major issue for us as we become adults, but it goes further than that. How we feel about our siblings can affect how we bring up our children and the life scripts we write for them which, if we're not careful, can lead to transgenerational difficulties.

As with all relationships in our lives, those with siblings are no accident. It's been said that we don't choose our relatives, but we do choose our friends. In fact, we choose them all. Those who are without siblings often mourn the fact that they're alone. Those who have siblings often wish they'd been an only child. Whatever—it is as it is and we have much to learn and discover from the family we chose.

What Helps Shape Love between Brothers and Sisters

It's generally expected that brothers and sisters will love each other. And of course they do—at least on some level, since we chose them just as we chose our parents as those who would help shape our early life. But sometimes relationships are difficult and the love appears to get lost in turmoil and pain. And where brothers and sisters are aware of loving each other, the manifestation of that love can be quite different for each child and unequal in its presentation.

There are many stages in the development of that love and things that affect it. Such as:

- the health of the family
- the expectations of the parents
- the parental relationship
- the innate temperament of the children
- the inner strength of the children
- family size
- birth order
- the sexes of the children
- the age differences of the children
- the presence or absence of parents

The eldest daughter who becomes a "little mother" to her youngest brother may appear to have a much greater depth of feeling for him than she does for another sibling. Brothers and sisters have their favorites, just as some parents do. Two children may enter into an alliance that isolates a third. As we'll see, children born early in a marriage have a different story than those born later and their development and capacity for loving each other may be affected.

The time gap between the birth of children is also significant. If for instance there's a particularly long gap between the birth of one child and another, or if the family has a broad age spread, the children will be separated by the point of development of their chakra system. For example if a child is developing his heart chakra (age 12 to 16) when a younger child arrives, his reaction to that child will be different to the power struggle that might develop if the elder child was still developing his solar plexus (age eight to twelve). With children who are born close together, for example if the second is born while the first is still developing the root chakra (under the age of three), different problems may arise. In this case, the elder child is still struggling with issues of survival which may appear to be threatened by the arrival of a younger sibling.

Twins or other multiple births present different issues, which will be discussed as a special topic later.

We all have problems—it's part of the human condition. Even in healthy families there are ups and downs. But it has to be said that some families just seem to function better than others (which is why they're often referred to as functional families). So before we look at what can go wrong, perhaps it would help to first have a look at what one of those model families might look like. Of course your family may have been very happy and be nothing like this—and that's fine. If the family you have now is different from this but happy, then just rejoice in what you have.

When the Family is Healthy . . .

Mom and Dad are happy together and in good health, as are the children. Everyone's aware of the love there is between them all, and though they argue from time to time, they always talk about what went wrong, patch things up and probably laugh about it later. They all know that they're securely held and belong together and that if anything were to go wrong, they'd be there for each other. They spend quality time together, eat and play together, though everyone has friends outside the family.

The parents set limits with love, and though the children try to push these now and then, generally they respect them. Sometimes they fight and have petty jealousies and rivalries, but they're actually very fond of each other and close ranks to protect each other if necessary. Feeling secure and rooted at home, they get on well with their peers and teachers, and perform confidently and well. In adolescence they may experiment a bit with behavior their parents might not approve of, but generally they know what's right and acceptable. They grow up to be good citizens with families of their own, learning to be good adults, self-reliant with good self-esteem and self-worth, from the example set by their parents and the other adults they know and respect.

Everyone knows that they can talk to each other about the good things and not so good things in their lives. They can bring problems into the open to be discussed and know that the family will stand by them even if not necessarily agree with their choices. There's mutual respect throughout the family. Special days are celebrated happily and there's joy and laughter and obvious love. In grief or sadness, they draw together to support and comfort each other. No one feels judged and there's mutual respect. When they go into the outside world, they carry an almost visible boundary around them that says, "We're family." They have a firm base for the rest of their lives.

One could say that these souls came together with little to learn from each other but with much to give in terms of nurture and love.

Does that sound like your family? If it does, great. But if not, don't despair. If you weren't so lucky, there are always things that can be done to heal where you are now.

The Not So Healthy Family

Some families are beset by a lot of pain and problems that cause the members of the family to have difficulties in relating to each other with a light and happy attitude. The family just doesn't function very well—which is why such families are often referred to as dysfunctional. In fact everyone is functioning to the best of their ability and is usually doing all they think they can do.

Mom and Dad probably came from families where there were similar problems and are doing their best to survive in the only way they consider possible. However, their inner pain may lead them to behave in ways that aren't conducive to everyone being able to relate in an open and straightforward way. Bringing up children and even staying together may be more than they can cope with.

In this family, relationships get a bit confused, communication is convoluted and everyone is touched by the pain in some way. Chronic stress, illness and unhappiness take their toll and drinking, drug taking, violence, abuse, neglect, criminality and separation are often part of the overall picture. The children of the family are invariably hurt (though often not intentionally) by the lack of security and the ongoing nature of the difficulties and their development—emotional and spiritual, and sometimes physical—is affected accordingly.

Sometimes the children parent each other. Sometimes they parent their parents. Sometimes they're parented outside the family for periods of time. But generally the children are much more aware of what's going on than parents give them credit for and they try to help by covering up, pretending, telling lies for their parents, looking after each other or bringing into play whatever other defensive strategy they can think of. Roles are confused and since security—or the lack of it—becomes a big issue, the children often cling to whatever they can to ride out the storm without drowning. Though often bonds are so flimsy that it's easy for family members to be thrown apart, for some, in an attempt to survive the turbulence, the bonds tighten to the point that they strangle normal development.

Since we depend on our parents for survival, with the ultimate terror being parental abandonment, either physical or emotional, as children we're willing to do whatever we can to protect our relationship with our parents at all costs and fulfill their expectations, no matter how sick or destructive they are. We juggle our own development with coping with an ever-changing landscape of parental emotions, competing for what little attention there is while trying to keep a sense of balance. It's not surprising that the scene is set for skewed

Guilt, shame and self-esteem

If yours was a painful family you may suffer guilt and shame, feel judged and criticized and have difficulties in coping with change.

Often guilt and shame get mixed up or are seen as synonymous. Guilt is a painful feeling of regret over something we've done, though we know it doesn't make us a bad person. Shame is a painful feeling about ourselves which results in low self-esteem and a feeling that we're of little value. Healthy self-esteem comes from the inside and even though we may feel anger, guilt or pain, or be criticized, it remains intact. If you have poor self-esteem you may feel worthless and blame yourself for things that are beyond your control. However, you might have defended yourself so much against the confusion you felt in childhood that your self-esteem has gone in the other direction: you feel that nothing is ever your fault and you find it hard to acknowledge that, like everybody else, you can make mistakes and that's okay.

relationships as we play out our reaction to the chaos with our brothers and sisters, often forfeiting the natural love and the relationship we might have had with them. Normal jealousies and rivalries may turn into deep-seated hatred, envy and resentment. Depending on what defensive strategy we chose to help us survive the chaos, we develop a pattern of characteristics that continues into adult life, marring not only adult sibling relationships, but those with others outside the family—friends, partners and colleagues.

Development of the chakra system can be damaged at every level if the problems within the family last throughout childhood, with deleterious effects on the developing personality. As adults we might have difficulty in making commitments and bonding, and are more likely to become codependent or have problems with intimacy.

In spiritual terms, members of dysfunctional families came together with much to teach and learn from each other, and are sorting out ancient associations with each other, repaying old debts and fulfilling ancient pacts and promises.

Don't despair! The good news is that once we're aware of what's going on, and why, we can start to heal our pain and change the relationships that feel stuck and sore. Of course we need to remember that we can only change ourselves and sometimes the other person in the relationship may not want to work as actively as you do. Still, on some level at least you can achieve resolution, as we'll see later.

Special times—special pain

Most of us have memories of special times we can look back on with happiness and share at family gatherings or tell our children about. But if your family wasn't a happy, healthy one, holidays and birthdays may have been times of increased pain. Unhappy, angry people can hardly rally and spend more time than usual together and enjoy it. Nor can they make a success of celebrating when the days before and after are abusive. Mealtimes may have been beset by arguments and worry, bedtimes delayed to try to prevent parental argument or spent hugging siblings and crying yourself to sleep. All this leads to distortion in spiritual and emotional growth. Such disharmony in the family continues to spill its poison throughout lives filled with pain and turmoil unless the issues are confronted and healed.

But true healing is a real possibility if you're willing to break the rules that you grew up with. These usually include: don't speak outside the family, don't trust outside the family and never tell anyone what's really going on.

Scary, requiring courage—but worth it!

Coping with Sibling Rivalry

Even in healthy families, difficulties between brothers and sisters occur, but these can be kept to a minimum by applying some sensible
strategies. Just like the parental pitfalls we looked at in the last chapter, if you can see yourself on either side, either as parent or child,
please treat yourself and everyone else with kindness and compassion. You and everyone else were doing their best in the light of your
understanding, information and development, so forgive where you
can. The meditation at the end of the chapter is there to help you.

Here are some simple precautions parents can implement to help
reduce sibling rivalry and jealousy:

- *Divide chores equally between the children (and particularly between boys
  and girls) and be aware of unfair responsibility falling on one child.* Often
  one child behaves over-responsibly and this develops into a
  lifelong pattern. Giving equal responsibilities and opportunities should reduce feelings of favoritism and jealousy and also
  prevent girls from growing up feeling like second-class citizens,
  subservient to men. Equality prompts their self-esteem.

- *Recognize their individuality and celebrate it.* Children who are dressed
  alike may look cute, but may hate not being allowed their
  individual style. Differences in talents and preferences should
  be respected. Anger about being deprived of their individuality
  is usually directed at the sibling who gets what he needs.

- *Be aware of the different ways in which they express themselves* and alert
  to what they might not be saying. Despite the fact that
  women tend to be more verbal in their approach to life, girls
  are more inner directed than boys, rarely revealing the
  intensity of their pain and anguish. Their self-doubt and the
  seriousness of their problems may be overlooked. Girls show
  their feelings by becoming depressed and developing problems
  such as eating disorders, whereas boys will "act out" more.

- *Allot equal importance to their futures.* The bright academic child
  needs to have the support of his parents with his future plans,

but perhaps even more so does the child who is less academic
and needs more attention to help him achieve his potential.

- *Be aware of their different rates of development.* Boys may lag behind
  girls in their development, but girls may also develop at
  different rates to their sisters. That goes for sexual
  development too. Teasing one child for being flat chested
  while the other blossoms is cruel and can set up feelings of
  inferiority that last into adulthood.

- *Spend time equally doing what they want to do as individuals.* It's
  difficult to give individual time to each child, especially in a
  large family, but it's time well spent. I know a family that goes
  rollerblading together every Sunday morning and swimming
  on Tuesday evenings. Sounds good? Yes, except that one little
  girl, Trudi, isn't athletically inclined and would love to paint.
  She rarely gets the chance to do that with her mom or dad,
  despite the fact that they're good parents who spend a lot of
  time with their children. Trudi is already jealous of her sister
  and brother and is not likely to tell her parents that. Her
  anger will eventually be played out with her siblings who
  already tease her for holding them back by falling off her
  rollerblades.

- *Give equal attention.* If one child is capable and dependable,
  giving little trouble, it's easy to fall into the trap of giving the
  other more attention.

Miranda grew up fiercely jealous of her elder sister,
Bethany, who was often in some kind of trouble and was
always being helped out by their parents. Whether it was at
school, at work or later in her marriage, Bethany had only
to whine and she'd be center stage. Bethany could prevent
her parents' attendance at Miranda's school play by being
unwell; ensure that every Christmas and birthday was
ruined by her dramas; get money in "loans" to pay off her
recurrent debts; have her mother talking on the phone till

midnight trying to sort out the latest drama in her marriage, etc., etc., etc. Occasionally their mother praises Miranda for never having given them trouble, but Miranda has never voiced her resentment in case that would put extra pressure on her parents, who are already tearing their hair out about Bethany. Both sisters are robbed of the possibility of closeness, partly because of Miranda's resentment at the unfair attention given to Bethany and partly because Bethany is so helpless and dependent that Miranda can't stand being around her. Miranda has little patience with other people in difficulty and though she's healthy and independent, she sometimes wishes she'd been less strong and well behaved: then she'd have gotten more.

- *Don't see one child as perfect*, and requiring little maintenance. This leaves the others feeling bad and less loved with lower self-esteem and self-confidence, which widens the gap further between them and the "perfect" child, to whom they react with anger, jealousy and even hatred. The "perfect" child may not be getting his needs met either since he will strive to maintain his position and deny his problems.

- *Be aware of the needs of a single girl among boys*. Often her needs are seen as less important and she may grow up angry, feeling subordinate to men, choosing relationships where she's submissive and allows herself to be used. She may well bring up her daughters in the same way. Of course the situation can be quite the reverse. The single daughter may be treated like a princess, with the whole family doting on how cute and sweet she is. This girl may grow up to be a prima donna princess who expects everyone to take care of her while she makes unreasonable demands on friends, partners and colleagues.

- *Be aware of the overprotective brother*. With the best intentions in the world, and with much love, older brothers may cripple their younger siblings by being too protective of them, fighting their battles (often quite literally) and preventing sisters from normal experimentation with boys because "no one's going to touch my sister." The brother grows up with difficulties, being overprotective of his partner and his children and stifling their growth.

- *Don't have a baby so that the older child will have a brother or sister.* Such arrangements usually backfire as both children grow up resenting the roles and expectations placed upon them.

- *Don't have another child to help hold the marriage together,* to keep a partner at home who might otherwise stray or to help curb the behavior of a partner, such as induce them to stop drinking. This sets up a host of expectations of the new child. The younger sibling may later be seen by the others as the one who sentenced them all to years more of misery when there was a point when they were almost free.

- *Don't displace an older child when the younger one arrives.* See Hayley's story, page 142.

- *Rid the family of myths.* If children are taught to lie to the outside world about what really goes on in the family, they grow up distrusting each other and those they meet in later life. Though discretion is a skill they will need (see page 72), learning to lie for their parents to protect the chaos results in them being unable to trust anyone. These children either rebel and leave or stay and collude, becoming a new generation of codependents who hide their shame and can never be themselves.

- *Be aware of what goes on in your home.* Incest is more common than we were once led to believe and this will be addressed as a separate issue in Appendix I.

- *Be aware that it's natural for you to react strongly to those children* who have similar personality traits to yourself. Though natural, it might not be good for that child or the others and might set up a current of rivalry between them.

- *Curb teasing.* It's been said that there's no such thing as a good tease. Though mild teasing may help children develop their

---

Ancient connections

On page 73, we talked briefly about reincarnation and past lives. If you would like to read a little more about this aspect of your present relationships with brothers and sisters and indeed other major figures in your life, then Appendix 2 may interest you.

---

tolerance and sense of humor and take themselves less seriously, it often develops into cruel taunting, sometimes to the point of abuse. The outcome can be a lowering of self-confidence, often with anxiety or phobia, to say nothing of the anger, whether internalized or displayed, that accompanies it.

- *Break up fighting.* Fighting might be part of the rough and tumble of life in some families, but some of the adults I see as clients were cruelly beaten by older siblings and weren't protected by their parents from this abuse. It's important that parents don't undermine one child in the eyes of the other by giving the impression that he needs protection: this widens the gap between them and leads to complexes that will spread to relationships with others outside the home. However, fights need to be broken up in a matter-of-fact fashion. Favoritism can lead a parent to turn a blind eye to the behavior of the preferred child, leaving her to run amok and terrorize the others—with detrimental consequences for the development of them all.

Breaking the Patterns of Our Childhood

It seems crazy, but as adults we tend to have a compulsion to repeat what has hurt us (see Hayley's story, page 142), actively selecting those people with whom we can play out the patterns again. Of course they're often doing the same thing.

If you came from a painful family, the likelihood is that you'll have become tolerant to inappropriate behavior from your brothers and sisters and your parents. You may have difficulties with boundaries —your own and other people's (see Mary's story, page 146). In adulthood you're likely to choose partners similar to your opposite-sex siblings or opposite-sex parent and to get hurt again and again in a repeated pattern before a major crisis forces you to look for help. Even then, you may find it difficult to take. You're more likely to give everyone else the benefit of the doubt, excusing inappropriate behavior while absorbing the pain, sometimes blaming yourself for things that are beyond your control and allowing yourself to be used and abused. You may also find yourself blaming everyone else for things that, in truth, are your responsibility. You may enable others to remain sick by telling lies for them, becoming the classic codependent enabler. You may be shocked to find yourself in the position of dealing out to others, including your children, some of the treatment you received and swore you'd never pass on to your children.

Often children within the brother/sister group fall into a particular pattern of behavior. You may see yourself and your brothers and sisters in the following descriptions, which are useful in predicting what strengths and weaknesses you might have as an adult and where you might want to do some work to make things better. The case histories, some of which need to span at least two generations, demonstrate just how far-reaching the consequences can be. You may have characteristics from more than one group.

Some families, on the face of things, seem quite "normal." But what's more important is how the children perceive what happens and how they react to it. Your feelings, whatever they are now, are valid. Please don't feel bad about however you reacted to your past. You'll find that as you start to look at how your feelings developed, and how they've pervaded every area of your life, they will start to change.

THE RESPONSIBLE CHILD

This child, often the first-born, tends to organize her brothers and sisters and everyone else. She can manipulate others into accomplishing what needs to be done and is capable, self-reliant, independent and a good leader. However, she's usually had little time to enjoy playing and being a child, and appears to have been a "little adult" for ever. As an adult she continues to take care of everything for everyone else and can be patronizing, bossy and meddling, enjoying sorting out others' problems whether they want her to or not. She's not much into feelings and doesn't like anyone to try to help her in any way. She can be detached and somewhat aloof, while underneath she's desperate for someone to acknowledge her. Does this remind you of anyone you know?

> Hayley was born, unplanned, a year after Tim and Jane married and the whole family was excited—the first child of the couple and first grandchild for both families. When her maternity leave was over, Jane returned to work, Hayley being cared for at a local nursery.
>
> Three years later, after a well-planned pregnancy, Thomas was born. Tim was overjoyed to have a son. By now he had been promoted, and Jane left work to be at home with the children, to return part time whenever she wished. After considerable discussion, it was decided that Hayley remain at the pre-school she now attended and where she was happy.
>
> Neither Tim nor Jane was prepared for the sudden change in Hayley's behavior. Usually a self-confident child, her performance at pre-school deteriorated. At home she became clinging, demanding attention. Jane responded to Hayley's behavior with exasperation, her patience being

tried by Hayley's tantrums when she didn't get her own
way. Thomas, on the other hand, was a smiling, cooing
baby, placid and easy and the center of everyone's attention. Though Tim made a conscious effort to "make the
children equal," it was obvious to all that Thomas was
the apple of his eye.

At 35, three years after the breakup of her four-year
marriage, Hayley developed a tranquilizer dependence.
Shortly after she and her husband parted she began having
panic attacks for which her doctor prescribed the
tranquilizer on which she was now dependent. She stated
that her ex-husband was a wimp who couldn't stand on his
own two feet. He'd always tried to please and appease her,
had been faithful and generous, but she ridiculed him for
the very qualities that many women would have loved.

Hayley was a difficult woman. Fiercely independent,
bossy and aggressive, she had a tendency to try to control
not only our sessions, but my behavior within them.
Whatever I suggested she claimed that she already knew,
and it seemed that she'd already decided that I could be of
no real help to her. Nevertheless, she continued to attend.

Hayley reacted strongly towards anyone who
appeared helpless in any way, and yet she gathered around
herself people who would be dependent on her and whom
she could control and push around. Eventually she hated
them for the very traits that attracted her in the first place.
As far as men were concerned, she knew that she gave them
a hard time. It was only when we talked about her
relationship with her younger brother that the source of
her problems finally revealed itself. Her whole demeanor
changed and her repugnance for him became obvious.

She remembered having been so excited that she was going to have a little brother and what it was like to see him for the first time and to touch him. But she recalled just as acutely feeling pushed out. Thomas's antics and his accomplishments had always been more important to her parents than hers. He had doted on his elder sister while she had little time for him. The more he tried to please her, the more contemptuous she felt.

At 19, Thomas announced that he was gay. Tim was visibly shocked and disappointed. Jane said that she could never accept it. Hayley stepped into the breach and discussed what they saw as a family tragedy with her parents and also gave Thomas the support he asked for. For a brief while they were close. Hayley felt useful and in control, though still detached from the suffering of the other three. She was so successful as family mediator that, after a few months, both parents changed their tune, began to accept the inevitable and took Thomas back into the family fold. Once again Hayley felt relegated to the sidelines, the good-looking, ever-smiling, charming Thomas back on his pedestal with their parents not only welcoming his friends home, but even being willing to meet his boyfriend. She felt sick and could hardly contain her jealousy. She was furious with him and even more so with herself.

The man Hayley married was tall, good looking, smiling and eager to please. Only now could she see how like her brother he was in many ways. She admitted that she'd controlled him for much of their brief relationship and was shocked to the core when he had the courage to leave her. Her fierce independence was shattered and the anxiety about being abandoned that she'd been feeling on some level ever since Thomas was born now surfaced.

She now needed to confront the jealousy she'd always denied and accept that it wasn't his fault that he was born the boy his father idolized, nor that he had a sunny personality that everyone loved. Hayley's anger was really with her parents, though telling them that would have risked further sidelining and loss.

A family session allowed her to tell the others how she'd felt all these years. They had seen her as independent, rejecting physical affection and being self-contained. Jane had been yearning for closeness between them and had substituted for the lack of this by finally accepting and loving the feminine side of her son. Thomas, having reluctantly given up on his sister long ago, was eager to have the kind of relationship with her that he'd always wanted, and they decided to spend some time together away from their parents to get to know each other.

It wasn't easy for Hayley to let go of her need to be in control and Thomas had to remind her that he was an adult with a life of his choosing and that he wanted her in his life as his sister, not a counselor. For Hayley, the renewed relationship with her family meant confronting issues of intimacy that she'd brushed aside for many years. However, as she did so, she began to soften and accept her own femininity in a way that she hadn't done previously. Her tendency to be the huntress in relationships subsided and the type of men she chose changed. Her anxiety and panic subsided and she reported that she had found not only her brother and her parents but also herself.

THE COMFORTER CHILD

This child takes care of everyone else's emotional needs. She's like a little therapist, perceptive, warm, empathic. A good listener, she soothes the hurt and disappointment of her siblings. As an adult she's always busy with other people's relationships, hurts and losses, though she rarely tells anyone about her own. She puts everyone's needs before her own and has problems observing other people's boundaries. From time to time she feels depressed, hurt and neglected, since her needs are rarely met, but she brushes those feelings aside and gets on with looking after everyone else. Sometimes she wishes that others could empathize with her, but if she was honest about her own difficulties she might feel diminished in their eyes. In any case she argues that if she had to *ask* for help, it wouldn't be worth having.

> Mary at 19 was one of life's grown-up comforter children. She was feeling hurt and confused, having had a disagreement with her roommate with whom she'd now parted company. She didn't quite understand what had happened, but on looking back, she was aware that there'd been increasing tension between them for the last few months.
>
> She and her friend Angela had got on so well that at the end of the first academic year they decided to move out of their college dorm and share an apartment. Mary was thrilled and did her best to take care of things, increasing her efforts when Angela seemed a bit irritable. A couple of months ago there'd been a slight disagreement when Mary, thinking that because they were so close her friend wouldn't mind, wore one of Angela's shirts without asking. Since then she'd been trying to please Angela by doing more and more. Recently, when Angela was away, Mary thought she'd surprise her by cleaning up her room. She was quite taken aback when Angela reacted with dismay rather than pleasure, said she didn't need looking after and asked Mary not to go into her room in the future. Now Angela had

decided they should no longer share the apartment. Mary was distraught.

Mary had grown up in a family where there was chaos much of the time, with unhappy parents who fought a lot about her father's heavy drinking. Her mother often complained of being tired and would go to bed, sometimes for several days at a time. The second child, but the oldest daughter, Mary had become adept at looking after the four younger children, ensuring that there was as little fuss as possible to take the strain off her mother.

With such a large family, there was little space or privacy. It was not unusual for Mary and her sisters and even her mother to share clothes and Mary had no idea that the lack of boundaries that she accepted as normal was not acceptable to other people.

What she saw as kind and caring behavior, indicating her close friendship with Angela, was actually intrusive. What's more, Angela had told Mary on several occasions that her behavior wasn't acceptable and had laid down limits that Mary simply ignored. In fact she misinterpreted Angela's messages and redoubled her efforts to please. Angela wanted a mutually respectful friend and housemate and Mary's behavior, which had been tolerable when they were friends living apart, had become intolerable given the intimacy of a live-in situation.

If you recognize some of yourself in Mary's behavior, perhaps you could think about being a bit more attentive to what others really want rather than making assumptions. You may have developed tolerance for inappropriate behavior yourself and have difficulty seeing why others find it intrusive. Though you may have been livid when a parent walked into the room and changed TV channels with no respect for the fact that you were already watching a program, you may find yourself unconsciously doing the same thing. Like Mary, you may feel shocked when others refuse to allow their boundaries to be crossed.

Learning to place boundaries appropriately (see page 154) and acknowledge other people's rights, while developing your own self-assertive skills, will help while you preserve your warm and loving gifts as one of the world's natural nurturers.

THE ACCOMMODATING CHILD

You may have responded to a confusing situation at home by not questioning what was happening, but simply keeping your head down and getting on as best you could. Accommodating children appear to be unaware of what's really going on around them. They make no waves, do as they're told, and like chameleons, adjust to the situation, detaching emotionally and losing themselves in books, daydreams or some creative pursuit. Their imagination is often their best friend. As adults, they may live in a bit of a fantasy world, which leads them to embroider the truth or frankly tell lies, unaware that their actions might hurt others. They drift along, agreeing to what everyone else wants, never stopping to question, take stock or make value judgements. They're kind, don't confront hurt, confusion or pain, and sometimes find themselves in situations they didn't quite expect, wondering just how they got there. Responsibility isn't one of their great assets!

Let's look at how Toby arrived at the point where he needed help.

Toby was a warm and sensitive, physically attractive young man and budding artist. Girls swarmed around him and somehow things had got out of hand. He really didn't know how it had happened, but he found himself simultaneously in relationships with two girls. This wasn't the first time he'd been in this situation, which ended in everyone including himself being hurt.

As a child, he generally preferred to be on his own, but he did remember snuggling his younger sister down in bed and telling her stories, a flashlight under the covers, when she was upset that their mother hadn't come home as promised to tuck her in. Toby had developed into a perceptive, empathic, creative young man, but he had little ability to focus, set boundaries and to say "No" when appropriate. He gained much of his self-esteem from his creativity, which girls in particular seemed to admire.

A light came on in his mind when he saw the similarities between his behavior with his sister and with the girls he attracted. He was being brotherly and affectionate, helpful and sharing his creativity with them, but as young adult women they interpreted his actions as something else and were naturally upset to find he was behaving similarly with others. His "help" was seductive and his hugs led to sexual encounters and an intimation of a commitment he didn't intend. Only when it happened a second time did he start to think that he might be the cause of it.

Neither Toby nor Mary had any healthy experience upon which to base their decisions and choices. If you see any of your own behavior reflected in their stories, then stop regularly, take stock and assess your behavior. Try to tune in to your body and feel your emotions. Discomfort in either area indicates that something's amiss. Asking yourself what's leading you to feel this will prompt you to assess whether your current behavior is acceptable. Look at whether there's mutual respect between you and others, and try to establish a set of healthy boundaries that will engender that respect. Being more open and honest with your friends and family about your difficulties will help, though do this with discretion. Most of all, check out what love means, since unintentionally you may be dispensing a brand that is damaging to you and others. Getting rid of your guilt that you weren't able to make everything right when you were a child will help you stop trying to do so now. It isn't your job to fix everything.

THE "ACTING-OUT" CHILD

Sometimes called the scapegoat, this child is perhaps the most courageous of all. He presents the whole family with an excuse for not looking at the real problems, since he's angry, often in trouble and bends his back to take the blows for all the family. He shows that things are painful and that not only he, but the whole family needs help, but often he does it so obliquely that his true message isn't heard. He's scared, though would never admit it; confused, though may profess to know it all; desperate for loving attention, but apparently rejects it, often attracting the opposite at home, at school and on the streets too. As an adult, he may have difficulties with impulse control, covering his sensitivity with drinking, drug taking or violence. He may be resentful that he was so busy trying to act out the problems of the family that he was labeled as a troublemaker, rejected at school and has never achieved his potential.

> Jess was bright, with a cheeky sense of humor and a good eye for a deal. He had a lot of business acumen and could have been financially secure. Women loved him and he appeared to have friends. He also had a cocaine habit.
>
> His brother Damian, three years his senior, had it all—a good job in the city, a snazzy car, expensive

apartment and lots of girlfriends. The only two children of a fairly well-off family, they'd had every possible material benefit bestowed upon them. They attended the same private school where, Jess admitted, he played the fool rather than getting on with his studies. At 15 he started to dabble with marijuana along with his friends and was politely asked to leave when found selling cigarettes laced with marijuana to younger boys. He returned home in disgrace and spent a couple of years at the local public school, where he was teased about his upper-class accent.

By the time he came for help at 31, Jess had a serious drug problem. Though their relationship had been strained for years, he'd called Damian and asked if they could meet. It was Damian who then took control of the situation, made the appointment with me, picked Jess up and drove him to the clinic.

Damian said that the last thing he wanted was that his parents should be alarmed by knowing there was a drug problem. He would deal with everything, and would ensure that Jess came to his appointments and complied with my recommendations. He talked of Jess as though he were a child and indicated that I should do likewise.

In fact, Jess needed little prompting to attend his sessions though initially he would rather joke than be serious about his difficulties.

Their parents had always been busy both socially and professionally and the children spent a lot of time being taken care of by a nanny or babysitters. When he was eight, Jess had walked into his parents' bedroom to find his mother there naked with a man he'd always known as Uncle Derek. He didn't even know whether they saw him, and he'd never told anyone. He did, however, start to wet the bed.

Damian had always been the good elder brother, achieving at school, getting along well with peers and parents, while taunting Jess mercilessly about his lack of development and his bedwetting, threatening to tell his friends. Jess's self-esteem and self-confidence had always been poor, his sense of autonomy almost non-existent. His love–hate relationship with Damian, with whom he simultaneously longed to have closeness yet feared, had been played out in a number of dependencies since. The fact that Damian had rushed into the breach now that Jess had admitted that he was in serious trouble filled him with inner conflict. On the one hand it was good to have his brother on his side, while on the other, he hated to give Damian anything else he could use against him.

My first step now was to get rid of Jess's collusion with Damian in not telling his parents about his drug dependency. This was a rerun of the bedwetting when Jess would do anything rather than have to feel shame in front of his friends. In fact, when they were informed by Jess himself of the situation, and that he was getting help, his parents were supportive.

The whole family began to sort out their relationships. Damian thought that he'd always taken care of his kid brother and that Jess had been very lucky because he, Damian, had had to make it by himself. Their father, never really present for his boys or his wife though loving them all, thought that the two boys had gotten along well. He felt he'd done the best he could for them by sending them to excellent schools and had felt equally proud of them both. Yes, he'd been shocked when Jess was expelled from school, but was proud of the way in which he then picked himself up and graduated, albeit a couple of years behind schedule.

Their mother appeared taken aback by the fact that there was a family problem. She was the younger sister of two brothers and there had been little focus on her as a child. She did well at school, loved to sit quietly reading while the men talked politics or science and now loved her job in the library where she could take care of the books, which she valued as almost sacred. She thought that her menfolk were getting on as those in her family of origin always had and that things were fine. Though Jess had had some problems in adolescence, she'd thought he'd grown out of them. She had a long-valued friend, Derek, who escorted her to functions since her husband was so busy. Her husband smiled and said Derek had been like one of the family for 20 years or more. Jess said nothing.

Jess at last began to look at his dependency and also to value himself. He had been a loyal son to both parents and a good brother, never giving a verbal hint to anyone about what he'd suffered, though it was all there in his behavior if anyone had cared to look.

This dynamic between the elder and the younger is not unusual. Sometimes there's such animosity that it's difficult to bring them together. The younger may remain stuck as a victim of bullying emotionally or physically and plays this out repeatedly in relationships with partners, colleagues and friends. Sometimes of course the child who has been bullied becomes the aggressor and later may resort to marital violence or physical abuse of his own children.

Do you recognize anything there? If you do, just be gentle with yourself. You've probably been covering your hurt with behavior that

Learning to set boundaries and limits

Healthy boundaries give us a sense of who we are, where we stop and other people start, what we're responsible for and what we can't hope to change. Though we'll be looking later at the fact that we're all joined spiritually, for the moment just imagine you have a boundary around the outside of your aura and that everything inside it is in your control, and everything outside isn't. Other people's behavior, feelings and actions are not things we can control. Boundaries protect us, help us to limit what we want coming inside that boundary, help us to be self-assertive and say no when we need to, and yes when we'd like to.

Now you can look at the things you don't want in your space, and following some simple rules, start to set limits with other people, lovingly, about what you want and don't want. The following example may help you.

One of my limits is that no one smokes in my house. Let's follow through some simple steps showing how I'm going to set and uphold that limit with love.

1. *I only take care of my feelings. Other people's feelings are beyond my control anyway, and starting to worry about them will just get me in a mess.*
2. *I know where the limit is and, whatever happens, it won't change. That doesn't mean that sometimes people are allowed to smoke in my house or that some people are allowed to. The limit is that no one smokes in my house.*
3. *Other people need to know my limit. It's unlikely anyone will attempt to smoke in my house, but if they do, I will say kindly but assertively that I don't like anyone to smoke in my house.*
4. *If someone overrides my limit, I need to know how I'm going to follow through. I will ask the person to take their cigarette outside.*
5. *If someone has overstepped my limit, I need to renegotiate with them in a different time and space. The next time they visit (if I want them to come back at all!) I'll meet them on the porch and remind them that there is no smoking in my home.*

you don't like for a long time. It doesn't have to be that way, though learning to live your life without some form of physical and emotional anaesthetic might not be easy at first. Try to talk to someone about how vulnerable you feel, leaving behind the bravado for a while. If you have to pick it up again now and then to survive, then so be it. But there needs to be a commitment to gradually living differently, otherwise achieving your potential and having the happier life you deserve will elude you. A word of caution—if drinking or using drugs has been part of the problem, your partner may also be having difficulties by now, so to expect them suddenly to change because you do may not be realistic. You may need to hold fast and prove your intentions before trust can be re-established.

How Birth Order Affects Us

The order in which we're born has a considerable bearing on who we become and how we relate throughout our lives. Not only does it affect our relationships with our brothers and sisters and parents, but it also influences our choice of romantic partners and the kind of expectations and conflicts we have with them.

THE FIRST-BORN

Parenthood doesn't come with an instruction book. The first-born is a living experiment for the parents. It's with this child that lessons are learned and mistakes are made. Sometimes those mistakes come in the form of being too lenient, but often it's the other way round and rules tend to soften with younger children as parents become more realistic in their expectations. The elder child has to break the ice, and often has less freedom.

If you were a first child, you may have been born at a time when your parents were less well-established financially and therefore had less materially. Perhaps, like Hayley's mother, yours continued to work, giving less time and attention to you than to subsequent children. While the first child may have come along too early and be resented in some way, the second child may have been planned and the stage is set with a different attitude. However, you may have been so eagerly awaited that all attention and expense was lavished on you in a way that wasn't possible for younger children. Perhaps you were also the first grandchild, so will always hold a pride of place that no subsequent child can match.

But being the elder, you probably shouldered more responsibility, and that may have made you bossy towards younger siblings, especially if they're of the same sex. If you're honest, you may like to control every scenario and gather around yourself others who will be dependent upon you. Do you have little time for anyone else's opinions? Undervalue other people's judgement? And get angry and jealous if someone else hogs the limelight? Often the older child feels competitive with the younger, especially as the gap between them closes and the younger catches up with the skills that have been admired as being special in the elder child. This may well lead the elder to withdraw angrily, refusing to be displaced. Do you recognize that?

Hayley subconsciously tried to sort out her problems with her younger brother by marrying someone like him. Sometimes two first-born children choose each other as partners because they have shared experience and understanding. However, there may be difficulties in adjusting to an equal partnership since both consider themselves to be the leader of the pack.

Of course you may be a very happy elder child with good relationships with all your family. I hope so. But if you're suffering, holding onto feelings of anger and jealousy that have been there for years, it's going to take you some courage to start to tell people how you really feel. Remember that it isn't your younger siblings' fault that they got what you didn't and your anger probably doesn't belong with them. Take care of your own needs and don't skip the rest of the chapter because it's important for you to try to understand how it may have been for your brothers and sisters.

THE YOUNGER CHILD

Were you the youngest child in your family? If so, you may have been more indulged and called upon to take less responsibility. You're likely to identify with your parents more than your brothers and sisters, and this alienates your elder sibling even more. You're probably fed up with always being told what to do and being bossed around and may have compensated by being sensitive to authority, having difficulty in taking instructions or working in a team and perhaps being a bit wary of those in charge, feeling inferior to them. You might become secretive about your behavior and hide your mistakes, fearful of criticism. This can make some younger children devious and dishonest. You may also have some difficulty with your sense of who you are and either tend to take yourself quite seriously (since no one else did when you were a child), or conversely never take yourself or anything else seriously because you're so used to having your opinion disregarded or overruled.

The relationship you have with your eldest sibling is likely to be difficult if they're of the same sex as you, as with Jess and Damian, or if the family dynamics were already askew. This can also lead to difficulties with same-sex colleagues. If you hero-worshiped your elder same-sex sibling, and tried to copy her and follow in her footsteps, there may be intense rivalry between you that continues into your adult life, even if it's never verbalized. The two of you need to talk about it!

If you have issues of resentment, dependency, submission or aggression, poor self-worth, and irresponsibility, you need to talk about them. If you're angry, jealous and resentful that older children escaped the misery by moving out and you were the one left behind to deal with warring parents again, you need to confront this and start to deal with your pain rather than letting it damage other areas of your life. There are some hints later on about how you might do that.

THE MIDDLE CHILD

The child who holds neither the special place of being the elder, nor that of being the "baby" sometimes gets lost and feels abandoned and rejected. Often this child feels mistrustful, with poor self-esteem and self-confidence and little identity. Is that you? Occasionally there are alliances between two of the children, leaving another, often a middle child, out, though this can occur with any combination of the sibling group. Parents need to take care that this child has her needs met, while not overcompensating and developing codependent bonds. Middle children tend to identify with one of the other siblings or the parents. In adulthood the middle child is often quite gregarious, dependent on approval from partners, friends and colleagues. However, they also have an easier time separating and eventually a better sense of their own individuality.

If you're a middle child, just be aware of your behavior with other people and see what you observe. Do you find yourself clinging to the outside of groups? Trying to join in where others are established in conversation? Do you find yourself hanging around trying to get others to say nice things about what you've done? Well, if you find you're doing that, then being aware is part of the answer to the problem. Give yourself the approval you need, start up your own conversations and see how scintillating you can be. You don't actually need anyone else to tell you you're okay. You are.

THE ONLY CHILD

Obviously there's no problem here with siblings, except that only children often long for some. If you are an only child be careful about looking for a parent rather than a peer in relationships. When two only children marry, they may have difficulties in sorting out who is to look after whom. Since sexual conflicts often erupt between partners who had no opposite-sex siblings, only children who marry each other may have difficulties in this area. If this is a problem for you, try talking to your partner about how it feels to you, and find out where each other's strengths and weaknesses are. Maybe till you feel more whole, you can each have specific brief times (like an evening or a Sunday) where one takes care of the other, as long as you do so fairly and make sure that you do for your partner what *they* like and not what you think they should like. Eventually you'll get to the point of caring for each other rather than taking care of each other. Your goal is to become your own loving parent.

TWINS AND MULTIPLE BIRTHS

There's something spiritually wonderful about souls who love each other enough to want to share the same womb. Whatever happens later, it's worth keeping that in mind. Some twins are close and so linked emotionally and spiritually that they know what goes on in each other's lives without needing to be told. Some are actually psychic, with telepathic powers, though usually these are confined to their twin unless further developed. Some twins spend much of their lives together, enjoying the closeness they had before birth and cherishing it throughout life. Some will even marry another set of twins. However, some twins are never happy to have been born as part of a duet, sharing birthdays and other celebrations and feeling that they never quite make it alone, and forever petition for their rights as individuals. Parents can help by not falling into the trap of dressing them alike, expecting them to go to the same places together, have the same friends and perform equally. Allowing them choice and celebrating their individuality will help keep rivalry to a minimum. It's

---

Incest

If this was a problem in your home you might like to read Appendix 1, which mentions some of the many texts that would be useful for you. No matter when this occurred, it's never too late to get help and to start to heal the pain and the difficulties you're still dealing with.

---

all too easy to refer to them as "the twins," "the girls" or "the boys" as though they came as a set and that's how they must stay.

With multiple births the blessings and the problems multiply, though parents of larger families tend to have a lot of help and counseling and are probably better equipped in some ways than the parents of twins.

Starting To Put It Right

Understanding how family dynamics affected not only you but your brothers and sisters can help you to open your heart and be more compassionate with them. However, even that may not blot out pain that you have carried for years. Sometimes at the death of a parent or some other major family event, siblings come together and start to search for the closeness that has eluded them for much of their lives. If you're now aware of how a problem with a brother or sister has been getting in the way of other relationships, it's time to try to put it right—even if you've tried many times before.

It takes courage and sometimes painfully hard work to tease out the strands that have enmeshed us and strangled what could have been good. For some, distancing and cutting off contact may seem the only way to deal with the pain. But that can become a negative template for how we deal with relationships, and in the end we may find ourselves isolated and lonely or hurtling down the path modeled by the family in the first place. In any case, we're bound to our source relationships forever no matter how far we distance ourselves emotionally or geographically.

With willingness on all parts, we can look back at childhood and see what really happened. What were the individual experiences of each child? Bear in mind your differences in temperament, how you were treated compared with each other and what your siblings suffered that you're only now aware of. It's not enough to say that you were all faced with the same conditions. If you find yourself in a painful relationship with a brother or sister, treat yourself (and them) with gentleness and bit by bit you'll be able to tease out what went wrong. It may be a while before you can feel warm and loving. As Antoine de Saint-Exupéry so eloquently put it, don't expect to plant an acorn today and sit in the shade of your oak tree tomorrow. But both of you deserve to have a loving brother or sister, so why not endeavor to find out what you chose to learn by being with them in this lifetime, then get on with the more creative bit of having a loving relationship. There's much more at stake than the sibling relationship itself.

Nor is it fair to blame parents for what went wrong with you and your siblings. Your parents were just working out their own problems as people while simultaneously trying to be parents, the only preparation for parenthood being their own childhood and what they gleaned from the families of friends as they were growing up.

Getting Back in Touch

If communication between you and your siblings has become painful, how about starting with a letter? Phone calls are sometimes intrusive, giving neither of you time to think and take a breath before being dropped into the pain that has caused disconnection. A letter can be prepared with time on your side and your sibling can also take time to read and re-read before deciding on their reply. Of course they may decide not to reply at all. That's their prerogative. But if you've made your move while being unattached to the outcome then your heart will already have started to soften and open and the pain may start to subside. It's great if the other party will come halfway, but if the pain's too much for them, if they've decided that distance is the only thing that works, if they're getting on with their lives and have managed to find some happiness, then that needs to be respected and you must set them free. Sometimes when you do that, on a high level there's a shift for both of you and the universe will give you a way to find each other again.

Sometimes this is just what was meant to happen in this life-time. If the two of you came together to play out the end of something begun long ago, then maybe you weren't meant to spend too long in each other's company this time. The connection is complete, the lessons learned and the two of you need to go your separate ways. If this could be so for you, simply send your sibling gratitude and love and send them on their way. The main thing is that you find some resolution to your pain and get on with your life accepting that things are as they are, and that there may be no more that you can do. Holding on to resentment and anger is only hurting yourself, so affirm to yourself as often as you can that you're letting it go.

Talking It Through

If the two of you are still able to chat about what went wrong and how you feel, then do that. Try to give each other time and space to talk without interruption, no matter how exasperating it feels. If one of you is likely to hog the time, you could always agree that each of you speak for a specific time. Another technique, originally used by the native Americans, is to have a speaking stick. It doesn't have to be a stick—any small object such as a feather or even a handkerchief would do. The person who's speaking holds it until they're finished and everyone else respects that and listens. When the speaker has finished, the stick is placed on the ground between you and the next person wanting to speak picks it up and holds it till they're finished. This may sound strange, but it's remarkable how it cuts down interruptions!!

If there have been serious difficulties and separation and you're lucky enough to get your sibling to a meeting, it should be in neutral territory rather than at either of your homes, and at a mutually convenient time. Try to prepare by letting go of resentment and anger before you get there. Of course you have a right to your feelings, and if you're resentful and angry, you have your reasons. But your siblings have their pain also and if they aren't at the point where they have as much insight and information as you, then it's up to you to take the high road and prepare the way with love. Not in a superior, patronizing or arrogant way, but with understanding. Read again what happens to your aura when you're angry and try not to take those vibes with you, since your sibling will sense them immediately. Their antennae have been primed by the same childhood as yours.

Sometimes it's better to invite someone else to the meeting as long as you both agree about this. This should either be someone who knows and cares for you both equally—perhaps an uncle, aunt or a mutual friend—or better still a therapist. Their function is to observe, to keep you on track, to refuse to take sides, but to reflect to you both what appears to be going on with you in the here and now. Sometimes they're also called upon to help you stay in the present and not revert to the anger that got you here in the first place. There'll be time for you to deal with that, hopefully, when the sting has been taken out of it by new understanding.

Be clear in yourself about your motives. Do you really want to put this relationship right or are you looking for yet another forum where you can have your say, blaming and casting up childhood memories of conflict and misdeeds by the other? If that's what you want,

Needs and wants

Sometimes it's difficult to separate these, especially if we've felt needy for much of our lives. I may want a new coat or to see a new film, or to have an evening out with a friend. However, my needs include being loved and nurtured (physically, emotionally and spiritually), having shelter, light and warmth, having clean water and good food, being of some service in the world and having a sense of my spirituality. If you come from a painful background, it's not surprising if you get your needs and wants mixed up. Sometimes you might feel very needy and dependent, or fiercely independent and willing to go without rather than ask for what you need. Sometimes you might be totally unaware of what you need or what you want. Or you may, because you feel bad about yourself, neglect your needs and not have what you want. Though often, for a variety of reasons, we have to go without what we want (and sometimes we're glad afterward that we did), we do deserve to have what we need. That means making changes in our inner and outer life to ensure that our needs are fulfilled.

then delay contact till you've come to terms with that childish desire and moved on to more maturity. Perhaps what's most important is to acknowledge that, for whatever reason, the two of you came together to these parents to learn something from each other and to give something to each other. If you're connected by only one parent, i.e. you're half-brothers or half-sisters, then the same applies. You've chosen each other and have a deep connection on a spiritual level even if you feel that was never realized in this lifetime. It can be very painful to yearn for that connection when the other no longer wants it, or perhaps never did. See that too with compassion for both of you. Yes, you've lost something, but so has your sibling in never really having had you.

The meditation that follows can be used at any time whether there is or isn't contact between you, whether you see each other and fight every day or whether you see each other but never really connect. Perhaps you could use it particularly to prepare for contact if there's been little or if it's been difficult.

Whatever happens, love yourself, be open to change and to new knowledge and information you didn't have before and be compassionate and empathic to the other. Let go of expectations, detach from the outcome and take it easy . . .

Affirmation

I open with love and forgiveness, to coming together spiritually with my chosen family. There is no separation between us and understanding flows between us on the highest level.

Meditation

Take yourself to your safe place and breathe deeply and relax. With every breath you breathe in, allow yourself to feel more peace and with every breath you breathe out let go of anxiety, anger, resentment and anything negative that is clinging to you and destroying your peace. You will see that a beam of white light surrounds you, protecting you.

Let light flow into the top of your head and as you feel yourself drift into a state of altered consciousness, take your focus down to your heart.

Gently breathe into your heart now and let it fill with green light. See your heart chakra spinning and spinning and opening, filling you with love and peace. Let the light coming in through your crown, divine light and love, flow down also, filling your heart. Enjoy the peace, enjoy the love and know that you are held gently and safely and that nothing can happen to you or damage you.

In front of you let your brother or sister appear. See them as a child, vulnerable and helpless as they once were no matter what has happened between you. Allow yourself to open with compassion to the events of their life, the pain, the sadness, the disappointments, the anguish, and know that both of you began in this same way with anticipation of a peaceful life with a love-filled future.

Be compassionate with yourself about what has flowed between you. Let love flow around the child self of your brother or sister and hold them in that light.

If you can, with love, send forgiveness for whatever has happened between you. There is no blame, no fault . . . Let it go. This child standing in front of you now is the embodiment of a great spirit just as you are. You may not know what brought them here, but they chose to be with you and you with them out of love for each other. Though that love may have become lost or distorted in this lifetime, it is still there at the level of your spirit. Feel it now. Let your siblings feel it too. Know that there is a deep connection between you which cannot be harmed by anything that has happened here.

Breathe love into the connection between you and say anything that you want to say to the spirit of your brother or sister. Hold them in this place of love for as long as you wish. Listen to whatever they may wish to say to you. Listen with an open mind and heart, allow yourself to receive whatever messages they wish to send. Be silent now and let the messages and insights simply drop into your mind, and trust that these are not of your imagination but are real.

Stay for as long as you wish and when you're ready, with a breath of love, allow your brother or sister to gently fade now and disappear, leaving you with the love for them and from them deep in your heart. Allow your heart to close a little, hold the light and the love and feel when your heart chakra is simply comfortable.

Focus again on your breathing and start to breathe into your arms and legs, to the tips of your toes and your fingers. Be aware of your physical being and love it. Feel your connection with the earth. Start to move a little now and when you're ready, gently open your eyes.

Stretch gently and have a drink of water, take time to orientate yourself, then take your journal and record what happened. End it with the affirmation that there is love between you on a spiritual level, that you are whole and so are they and that you send them love and light for the higher good of you both.

Seven

The Love of Friends

*No medicine is more valuable, none more efficacious, none bet-
ter suited to the cure of all our temporal ills than a friend, to
whom we can turn for consolation in time of trouble, and with
whom we may share our happiness and joy.*

—AILRED OF RIEVAULX

Friends come to us as gifts from heaven, and friendship as a
sweet grace that enriches us and helps us enjoy our lives as an
adventure of the spirit. True friendship is one of life's greatest treas-
ures, which can lead us to levels of understanding and depths of communication we may never have envisaged. Good friends stimulate us
to develop and unlock those hidden parts of ourselves we'd hardly
recognized and to express them to the world. They stand beside us
at occasions of joy and crisis offering us love and comfort which, at
times, possesses an intimacy beyond the sexual intimacy of partners,
the protective passion of parents or the expected love of siblings.
Chosen friends occupy a unique place in our lives and hearts. It's to
them that we often reveal more of ourselves than to any other, since
the tie between us is different, and the expectations too. We're bound

by neither blood nor law, free to come into each other's lives and to leave, or to stay forever, through a lifetime and beyond.

What Makes a Good Friendship?

It's been said that the perfect friendship is the deepest and highest sentiment of which we're capable. Certainly it's a major factor in our emotional health and happiness, a force sustaining both parties, a potent catalyst in our mutual growth, which lends a lightness and joy to life. It encompasses an unselfish desire for the other's well-being, for their genuine good, their health, their happiness and the achievement of their potential. The purity of love that flows between friends is a truly spiritual experience for both. It's the recognition of the inner divine of the other that prompts the selfless giving of something of our soul to our friend.

Mutual esteem is essential to the good friendship. As one friend complements the other, both are inspired and ennobled as they happily accept, appreciate and reciprocate the sweet delight of the friendship. Mutual sharing on several levels is also a natural part of friendship, though men and women may differ in the quantity and quality of the exchange. As trust in the love and confidentiality of the friendship develops, vulnerability diminishes and less is withheld. Willingness to have honest and deep communication is the hallmark of a mature friendship, revealing to our friend those parts of ourselves and our lives that are not generally in the public domain, as well as the more frivolous aspects. Such honesty allows us to relax, play, laugh, have fun, express our feelings and be comfortable being ourselves whether we feel strong or vulnerable, competent or filled with self-doubt. We know that any flaws of behavior or character we reveal will be accepted, handled with gentleness and will not be used as weapons against us. We need neither to hide nor flaunt our power, knowing that our friend will continue to respect us, love us and wish us well no matter what. The thoughts, feelings, beliefs, joys and sorrows, desires and choices shared in friendship connect us, heart and soul.

Though the desire to share time and gain pleasure from the friendship is natural, if the relationship is motivated either by self-aggrandizement or potential gain, its authenticity is questionable.

For some, friendship almost replaces family, giving us a similar sense of security and continuity.

Making Friends

Friendships don't come into our lives fully fledged, but are built over time as we talk to each other and listen, sometimes for hours at a sitting, revealing more and more of ourselves, taking risks in being honest about who we are, sharing more and more deeply, until we're intuitively aware of each other's needs, sensitivities, loves and fears. But sometimes, like falling in love at first sight, there's instant recognition, attraction and appreciation, and we know that here is a friend for life. As John O'Donohue in *Anam Cara* puts it, "This friendship is an act of recognition and belonging." It may be that we recognize this person as someone we have known much longer than this lifetime.

From a multitude of acquaintances we might choose several we call friend, but in a lifetime we're lucky to have a handful of friends with whom our hearts are truly in tune and with whom we can be comfortable and at home.

To gain a friend we need to be a friend, and that means being willing to give of ourselves, our time and our love. As we develop as individuals, the way in which, and the reasons why, we choose our friends change. In the past when we were more rooted as a society people tended to make friends in childhood and keep the same friends for life. Friends were almost an extended family. As time has gone by and we are more nomadic in our lifestyle, we have diversified our friendships.

In early childhood we make friends with those who are readily available—in our class at school or living in our neighborhood. As adolescence approaches, and with it greater mobility, friends are selected more carefully from those with common beliefs, interests and shared experiences, and generally are those with whom we're socially and academically compatible. In young adulthood, similar interests, whether family, political, philosophical, religious or spiritual, draw us together, and some of these friendships last a lifetime. Adult friendships tend to be with those with similar lifestyles—women often find themselves making friends with women with children of similar ages, while men make friends with those who have similar hobbies, or with colleagues at work. Mature friendships are often those made earlier in life, but new friends are those with similar philosophies and lifestyles. In old age, when once again mobility may be restricted, new friends are again selected from those who are available.

Though usually there must be some similarity in personality, background and lifestyle for a friendship to spring up, friends may come to us in unexpected ways, occasionally the most unlikely people becoming firm friends. We may have known someone for a while before the spark that ignites friendship is kindled at exactly the right time for both of us, and friendship is born. It's wise to remain open to the opportunity of friendship at every moment and in every place.

Opening Our Hearts in Loving Friendship

Opening our heart chakras and forming a bond is what prompts the development of friendship and sustains it. Giving each other strokes in the form of attention, approval and affection; demonstrating love with a touch or a hug; showing compassion and that we appreciate the sense of connection with each other sustains us through the normal ebbs and flows of friendship. As in any other relationship, if, because of jealousy, anger, resentment or anything else that forms a barrier between us, we cease the flow of love, our heart chakra closes and the link between us becomes tenuous and eventually breaks.

Sometimes we naturally outgrow each other as our attitudes and interests change. Occasionally, though a friendship may be deep and meaningful, it is brief and there follows no contact, but the relationship has nevertheless changed our lives forever and the love between us lasts on some level. Some friends never meet, drawn together only by the written word, enjoying a lifetime of shared intimacy and deep friendship in letters spanning years. Neither the length nor the frequency of contact is as important as the spiritual connection, though most of us yearn to spend time with our friends, since that is part of the loving. For good friends, neither time nor distance can touch the love and sense of belonging. You can slip back into the comfort of being together no matter how long you've been apart.

From the time of acquaintance, friendship develops when, though the talking is stimulating and fun, the silence between the two of you feels comfortable too. Mutual trust and loyalty develop, with a sense of give and take. Friends learn to respect and accommodate their differences. Closeness develops. Though there may come a period of boredom and stagnation, when the relationship is tested, true friendship will survive and become stronger. Where friendship is not truly established, it may self-destruct at this point. One may start to find fault with the other and conflict may develop. This either resolves with the dawning of new respect and understanding, or else this is the time when the friendship falls apart. No matter how deep and special a friendship, it often goes through ups and downs, arguments and reconciliations, though the more mature we become, the less obvious they are.

Are You a Good Friend?

- Are you willing to love them enough to risk their anger or rejection?
- Can you put yourself in your friend's shoes to see how it feels?
- Are you willing to challenge destructive behavior for the good of your friend, but without being judgmental?
- Are you able to be as honest about *your* feelings as about *her* deeds?
- Are you willing to reveal yourself?
- Are you open to forgive and let go of things once they are resolved? (Forgetting might be impossible, but forgiving is essential.)
- Do you cherish your friend's secrets and confidences?
- Do you share in her hopes and delight in seeing her grow?
- Do you always try to have a positive attitude and look for the blessings and joy in every situation?
- Do you listen with understanding and without judgement, without offering advice (unless you're asked for it) or trying to fix things, and show interest and appreciation?
- Do you apologize when you know you were wrong?
- Do you give your friend space? (An old saying is that friends are lost by calling often and calling seldom.)
- Are you supportive but willing to stand back and just be, allowing your friend to find her own way to salvation? (Often just knowing you're there is enough.)
- Do you give encouragement and cheer your friend on even if that means she'll overtake you?
- Do you sometimes bring flowers or a little token of your friendship or of commiseration or joy?
- Are you willing, when necessary, to give a firm tug to get your friend out of "poor me" mode and back on track?
- Can you refrain from saying "I told you so"?

Or . . .

- Do you try always to be "nice" rather than being honest?
- If you are honest, is it really for the good of *both* of you or just to let you vent your feelings?
- Are you perceptive enough to choose with care your time to be honest or just blurt it out whenever you want to?
- Do you cover up conflict and pretend it's not there, and thereby prevent true intimacy from developing?
- Do you refuse to handle disagreements honestly?
- Do you avoid dealing with issues then talk behind your friend's back?
- Are you able to temper honesty with kindness?
- Do you criticize and correct? (See Rita and Sandra's story, page 176.)
- Do you take without asking or forget to return what you borrowed? (Remember Mary? See page 146.)
- Do you take up more than your fair share of the time with your problems or your good news?
- Are you demanding or bossy?

What Can Go Wrong?

Of course there are innumerable things that can go wrong, but we'll look at only a few of them here. Since good intimate communication is essential, so are confidentiality and respect, the betrayal of which can damage the friendship severely.

NOT BEING HONEST ABOUT OURSELVES

Sometimes it takes a while before there can be enough trust in the relationship for honesty to be part of it—and so it should. All of us have learned to hide parts of ourselves and be somewhat secretive about our inner lives. The boundaries of those who appear to dash headlong into frank disclosure are often a little suspect. Until the friendship deepens, it might be too scary for each of you to reveal much of your inner self. But in a way that's a Catch 22 situation, since it's only by taking the risk of being open that intimacy can develop sufficiently to allow further trust to grow. If you're perceptive you'll know when to be discreet and when the friendship can cope with a bit more disclosure. One thing's for sure: if you want the relationship to last, there needs to be a time when you're both willing to get beyond "nice" and into the honesty that the intimacy of long-term friendship demands.

Becoming honest about who we really are can be a painful process as we start to recognize our not-so-nice bits—what might be termed our shadow—but until we do, we aren't complete. Sometimes it's friends who help us acknowledge and accept that part of ourselves.

NOT BEING HONEST WITH OUR FRIEND

Often we find it harder to be honest with our friends than with strangers, especially if what we need to say is something the other person may not want to hear. But being "nice" rather than honest is neither loving nor kind. Our friends deserve more from us than that. Of course we look for times of fun, laughter and shared joy together, but being a friend is also having the courage to confront issues in a way that others don't dare to do or don't love enough to do. Often in psychotherapy groups, when encouraging members to be honest with each other, I've said that anyone can say the nice things, but it takes someone who loves us to risk saying the things we might not like to hear. It's worth remembering that when someone confronts us.

Talking behind your friend's back, breaking confidences and sharing their secrets are all forms of dishonesty that dishonor your friend, yourself and the person to whom you gossip. Think about the damage you can do with careless words to which someone else adds their own interpretation before handing them on. You have no control over what happens next, but your dishonesty towards your friend has damaged the trust between you and the betrayal can hang heavy for a long time and may never be completely resolved.

CORRECTING AND COACHING RATHER THAN SHARING FRIENDSHIP

Have you ever had one of those friends who rushes in with advice and is always trying to "help" by telling you where you went wrong and how you could have done it better? Who, for our own good of course, is always telling us how to do it—how to drive better, to cook, to brush our teeth, to deal with other friends? Though the motive may be pure, the damage to both parties is inevitable. Do you sometimes do that? This is often where our source relationships start to raise their heads in our friendships.

Sandra and Rita met quite by chance, or so it seemed. Sandra was returning from attending a seminar on caring for the elderly in her capacity as a welfare worker in the community. Rita was returning from visiting her mother. The train was full and they were seated together and got into conversation. They were both in their early forties and immediately felt that they had much in common despite the fact that they had quite different lives—Sandra was living alone and working full time, Rita was bringing up her 12-year-old and sorting out their new home since she and her husband had recently moved into the area. Finding that they lived relatively close to each other, by the end of the long journey, they decided to meet the following week for lunch.

Friendship blossomed quickly. Rita had been so busy that she'd almost forgotten the joys of having a close friend living nearby, and her husband was supportive of her taking time to spend an evening a week with Sandra. Sandra had been focusing on her career and though she had some long-term friends, she felt close to Rita and looked forward to their evenings together. However, even though they felt they had much in common and liked each other, it wasn't long before Rita started to feel a little uneasy about their meetings. She couldn't quite figure out what was wrong until on one occasion she caught herself slightly altering an anecdote she was telling Sandra, and with a tight feeling in her chest, realized that this was exactly what she'd learned to do with her elder sister.

Over the next few weeks she carefully observed just what happened between her and Sandra, marveling that she hadn't noticed before—but then why should she? It was exactly what she'd grown up with. It seemed that when she revealed something about her life to her friend, Sandra usually had some helpful comment to make: a remark about how Rita could have done it differently, what she should have said, what Sandra would have done under the circumstances, how Rita should proceed now. Sometimes when Rita was admitting where she had gone wrong, Sandra would not only agree but leave Rita feeling foolish, to the point where she wanted to hide some of the truth rather than risk Sandra's disapproval. When Rita had shared a new skill she had learned, rather than simply enjoying her achievement, Sandra told her how it could be better still in a rather superior and patronizing way. Though sometimes it was fairly subtle, Sandra had taken it on herself to constantly correct Rita.

In fact, Rita was the younger of two sisters, and though as intelligent as her sibling, she had been criticized and corrected and still felt less worldly and informed than her sister. Though she and her sister now had a tenuous relationship, Rita still thought of her, even in adulthood, as her big sister who knew best. Sandra, on the other hand, was the elder of two sisters by several years and she felt her sister still needed her care and protection as she always had done. Sandra and Rita had recognized this in each other and it was this similarity that had brought them together as friends (see Chapter 8). Luckily both were honest enough to confront the issue gently and salvage the friendship, though Rita remained wary for a long time until she also began to confront her sister.

This tendency to give unasked-for advice, to meddle in the lives of others and to present ourselves as a helper when what's asked for is a friend, is destructive, no matter how well meaning. Even if someone does need help, this high-handed approach, which indicates that we think we know better than the other person how to live their life, is hurtful, undermining and discourages our friends from being honest with us or asking us for what they need.

Unless we understand it and confront it, this tendency to bring our past into the present can damage even the best of friendships. Sometimes friendships end not because of what is actually happening but because of what we expect will happen. We tend to respond more to the distorted image from the past in which our present friend had no part. Sometimes it's only when intimacy starts to develop that we become aware of somehow having been in this place before and having been hurt and this causes us to retreat, at times with a display of childlike behavior.

ALLOWING OURSELVES TO BE USED

Sadly there are some who take advantage of our friendship and use and abuse us. If we're either too nice to say no or too afraid of the consequences if we do, we can get caught up in all sorts of difficulties. If you find a new friend who is very open, then be wary since openness usually develops over time and discretion in the early phase of friendship bodes well for the future. If you feel drained and helpless after spending time with your friend, then you really need to look at what's happening. We talked on page 17 about energy exchange and how some people take our energy without being aware of doing so. However, some people are well aware of what they're doing and allowing it to continue isn't helpful to you or them.

People like Mary (see page 146) have problems with boundaries. They may be inconsiderate and make long, demanding phone calls late at night or at other inconvenient times. There may be veiled threats as to what might happen to them if you don't listen, if you withdraw your support or are not there for them. There may be even more frank emotional blackmail. They may seem to listen to you, but start the next sentence with "Yes, but . . ." With this person, you're getting nowhere. In fact, the longer you allow the manipulation to continue, the more you're increasing the problem. The person will become more and more dependent upon you (which may feel nice in the first place but will soon wear thin) and will simply get worse since you're rewarding their bad behavior with more attention.

Another way in which friends can use you is to deny what they're really saying or doing, asking you to collude with them. This happens for instance when someone makes a snide remark and then denies it, or when your friend gives you the cold shoulder but insists that they're doing nothing out of the ordinary. It's important that you go with your intuition. Truly listening with your ears, eyes and heart will reveal much more than is in the words.

The kindest and most loving thing you can do is to be honest with them about what you perceive and insist that they stop using you in this fashion. This self-assertive approach is being a good friend, even if the other person doesn't think so. You can still talk to the healthy part of them if you want to, but make it clear that if they stray down the path of manipulation, you'll end the conversation. This also goes for people who want you to listen to their gossip and ask you to take sides against other friends. You can always continue with the friendship on these terms if you want to while your friend learns a more healthy and loving way of being with you.

BEING DRAGGED DOWN BY NEGATIVITY

Sometimes people are so negative that it's painful to be around them, and allowing them to drag you down and fill your atmosphere with negativity is not good for either of you. If this is a new development in your friendship, perhaps you could gently explore what has happened in your friend's life to lead him to be bitter and cynical. I'm not suggesting that you desert your friends in time of trouble, but if you have a friend who's constantly negative, ask yourself what you're gaining from the friendship and why you chose this person to be your friend. Lovingly confront her and share your exasperation. Sometimes negativity is a learned behavior (someone in the family may have demonstrated this), and can be unlearned and replaced by a more positive outlook. Are you gaining something from being able to be a rescuer here? Perhaps your friend is depressed (and you may be too) and should be properly assessed to see if he needs professional help. There's a checklist of symptoms of depression in Appendix 3.

SELFISHNESS AND INSENSITIVITY

Jacqui was fed up with Lee and even though they'd been friends since schooldays, the friendship was at present somewhat strained. Bright and bubbly with a great sense of humor, Lee had always been loved by everybody—especially the men they knew. She was cute, playful and charming and that was part of what Jacqui loved about her. She was always the center of attention, which most of the time was okay.

Married for three years, Jacqui was pregnant for the first time and really thrilled about her news and how special she felt. She'd been longing to tell Lee, and when they met for their usual Thursday evening while Jacqui's husband and Lee's boyfriend were off bowling, she was bubbling with excitement. She was astounded and not a little hurt when Lee said a quick "Congratulations," gave her a brief hug, and launched into the latest office gossip, with Lee as the star of course! What was even worse was that Lee appeared oblivious to the fact that Jacqui was hurt, despite her quietness for the rest of the evening.

This wasn't the first time that Jacqui had been hurt by this kind of thing, but as usual she said and did nothing—and nothing was going to change until she did.

This kind of selfish insensitivity can ruin the best of friendships, and though we may make excuses for our friends and just put up with their selfishness, other people won't. It would therefore be kinder to Lee if Jacqui confronted her about her behavior.

DEMANDING FRIENDS

Friends make time to be there for each other, to listen to and comfort each other, and yet they understand the demands on the other's time and understand when other things in life must take priority for a while. They believe in each other's judgement, respect each other's pain and know that, though there may be cycles of closeness and distance, their emotional and spiritual connection always brings them back together to share in the love between them. Sometimes jealousy about others taking up our friend's time and usurping our position as their special friend threatens the lightness of the way in which we hold each other.

Marjory was having a difficult time. Her parents had recently divorced and she was not only trying to deal with the huge upheaval in her own life, but was trying to support her 16-year-old brother, Scott, who wasn't coping very well. She was trying to make it comfortable for him to choose to be at her apartment some nights to take a break from the heavy atmosphere at home, and also to give her mother time and space to do her grieving without having to worry about Scott.

It had been a difficult six months and she was aware she hadn't spent as much time as she used to with her best friend, Beryl whom she used to see most days. They would pop into a bar on the way home from work, have a quick glass of wine together, and a couple of nights a week would get take-out and take it to either of their apartments and watch a video. All that had changed, though Marjory still tried to see Beryl once a week alone. She invited her over sometimes when Scott was there and suggested that the three of them go to the movies occasionally. They also talked on the phone regularly.

She'd been so wrapped up in her problems that she'd hardly noticed Beryl's cooling off until a fight erupted one evening when she called.

She was quite taken aback by Beryl's fury and demands that she get her priorities sorted out. Beryl said she felt that the friendship meant nothing to Marjory and that unless they could spend time together as they used to, she wanted no more to do with Marjory.

Though Marjory could sympathize with Beryl, who had obviously been more dependent on the friendship than she had, she was hurt that Beryl was demanding what she couldn't really give right now. In fact, Marjory herself needed understanding and loving support from her friend. Though they managed to patch up their friendship, Marjory was left feeling that the freedom and support she had thought were mutual in the relationship were just an illusion.

When there is too much intensity in a friendship, one tends to focus on the other and demand closeness, time or exclusivity. Usually such demanding behavior is caused by jealousy and insecurity. Often the only way the other can deal with this increased pressure is by distancing, leading to further polarization and escalating demands, as the friendship becomes more and more fraught and unmanageable.

UNWILLINGNESS TO FORGIVE

Perhaps one of the most damaging things in any relationship is the unwillingness to forgive and let go. It would be a strange relationship if there was never a time when friends hurt each other. That's part of the growing process and part of what in the end strengthens both us and the friendship. Learning about ourselves as our friend reflects things we might not like and challenges us to change, is bound to leave us in pain at times. If the friendship is secure and based on love, it can absorb such trials as each friend knows that, in the main, they are accepted for who they are. Forgiveness is a choice. We can choose to hold on to our wounds and nurse them—and that might be acceptable very briefly—but in the end, being willing to forgive is the only road to peace and happiness in any relationship. Without it your friendship will founder and eventually die.

RESCUING RATHER THAN BEING A FRIEND

If you find yourself repeatedly doing things for your friend that she could do for herself, if you find yourself constantly denying your friend's self-denigrating comments; if part of your function as friend appears to be to bolster a flagging ego, then you're probably in a rescuing game that can only lead to dependence and resentment for both of you. It may feel good to be the one to give advice and help keep your friend on track, and to know that you're the one they choose to tell all their troubles to, but every time you allow your friend to use you in this way she becomes more dependent and in the end feels inferior to you, helpless and lost while you appear to gain in superiority. If you allow someone to play this powerful role in your life, beware! Have the courage to take back your power even if that means you have to struggle a bit to find your feet again.

> Katy comes from a chaotic family and her self-esteem has never been good. She could hardly believe her luck when Anne befriended her. They seemed to have some things in common, but Katy, from the beginning, saw Anne as being much more worldly than herself. It was great to have someone around who was so helpful and kind. Anne had also had a difficult childhood, though she didn't share this with Katy.
>
> Katy was overwhelmed by a deluge of paperwork associated with her divorce and was feeling vulnerable and in a bit of a panic about it. When Anne came over one evening she kindly offered to take care of some of it, which she did. Katy was relieved and grateful. She was

overcome with gratitude when Anne offered to drive by the lawyer's office the next morning and drop off the papers so that Katy didn't have to worry about them any more.

As the date for the court hearing approached, Anne was more and more helpful, and Katy, stifling uncomfortable feelings of embarrassment at taking up so much of Anne's time, thanked her profusely. When Anne suggested that she'd take time off work and come to court to offer her support, Katy was full of gratitude and love for her friend. As the day approached, Anne coached Katy in what she needed to say and do, but for the first time Katy felt a little uncomfortable since some of the things Anne proposed were not quite what she'd had in mind. There was a touch of irritability in Anne's voice when she responded that she was only trying to help and of course she would withdraw and leave it all to Katy if that was what she wanted. Katy felt some of the old panic arise in her chest at the thought of having to cope alone, and suddenly realized that she knew very little of what was really going on because she'd allowed Anne to do so much for her that it was Anne who was really conversant with the case.

On the day of the hearing, Anne picked Katy up to drive her to court, having already said that she knew it would be a difficult time for Katy. A pre-hearing meeting was arranged with Katy's legal representatives and Katy asked that Anne, her best friend, might sit in with her. She was taken aback when Anne started to make points to the lawyer on her behalf and even argued with him about the advice he was giving to Katy. She found herself feeling small and helpless, nervous and out of her depth even more than she used to.

In the days following the hearing, Katy wanted to have some space and time to think and grieve. She felt confused and lost and, for some reason, angry with Anne. She didn't blame her for anything, but she still had an uncomfortable feeling that there was something going on that she didn't quite understand. She made an excuse when Anne called to come over, but by the second phone call, Anne was irritated and demanded that she come over to see if Katy was all right. No amount of gentle dissuasion was working so eventually Katy agreed, adding that she was tired and wanted to have an early night.

The evening was not pleasant. There was a change in the way in which Anne spoke to her, and finally, when Katy insisted that she needed to rest, Anne blurted out that she was very disappointed in Katy and that after all she had done for her, she didn't expect her to behave like this. Filled with guilt, Katy apologized and made another cup of coffee and the two sat on into the late evening discussing what had happened in court and how Katy felt now.

This is a classic rescue situation where the "friendship" is based on a power gradient with Anne taking the high road and leaving Katy feeling more and more helpless, inferior and lacking in skills, while Anne becomes more powerful, assuming a position where she can be Katy's righteous persecutor if she steps out of line, and can also play the victim of the piece if Katy should object. Sadly, not being fully aware of the game, Katy falls back into it and allows more and more rescuing, getting herself deeper and deeper into a hole.

At the beginning of the transaction, Anne probably offered help with a good heart. But in the end it was neither help nor friendship she gave. Real help might have included Anne sitting beside Katy being supportive, while Katy dealt with the paperwork herself, a process in which Katy would have learned what she needed to know in order to deal with it competently. She would have developed new skills, which would have been good for her self-esteem, and Anne would still have had the joy of knowing that she'd helped her friend. As it was, by the time they reached court, Katy knew so little of what she needed to know that Anne was able to undermine her authority and take over, leaving Katy looking and feeling rather foolish and out of touch. Katy's gratitude for the amazing amount of "help" that Anne was giving her prevented her from telling her friend to back off and give her space when she knew that was what she needed. It was obvious to Katy by then that such behavior would be interpreted as ungrateful and petty and she didn't want to offend the person who had been so very kind. And so she was caught in the web.

This kind of rescuing behavior, which seems on the face of things to be ultra kind, is not about friendship, but dependency. With every rescue, every attempt to do for us what we would happily do for ourselves, there is the subconscious message that this person could actually live our life better than we can, and a state of irritation and learned helplessness and resentment set in. In fact in this case Anne is the more dependent, since she needs the kind of gratitude and adoration which Katy so freely gave, along with the power to control. One must also ask what's really going on in Anne's life for her to need to disempower others in order to feel empowered herself.

ALLOWING YOURSELF TO GET LOST

It was Eleanor Roosevelt who said that unless we're a friend to ourselves, we can be friends with no one in the world. Allowing ourselves to become subsumed in the friendship till our own identity is lost leaves us with little to offer. Try to keep a clear picture of your own beliefs and philosophies, though of course these need to be flexible and open to change when there is a good reason to do so. It's fine, and even enriching, for there to be differences between us. We don't always need to agree and forget who we really are and what we think. In losing your sense of self, you cheat both yourself and your friend too.

Sometimes we get lost in the other's generosity, which can become intrusive and even aggressively suffocating despite the fact that they have the purest of motives for almost forcing this upon us. It's both demoralizing and undermining, especially if one person has difficulty in reciprocating the generosity or the other refuses to accept generosity in return. The one who is being drowned in a sea of generosity will always on some level feel inferior to the other and never be able to find themselves or their place in the relationship.

THINKING OUR WAY IS THE ONLY RIGHT ONE

If we believe that our way is the only right one and that we're the only one to perceive the reality, then we intimate that everyone else is wrong in their interpretation of events. Such rigidly held views can then become obstacles to closeness, with resultant anger, isolation and anxiety and a breakdown of the friendship. With an open heart and mind, there's always much to learn. What we perceive from our viewpoint may be very different to the perception of the same thing by someone with different life events, background, religion, culture, sex, age and tradition. Even though we're most likely to choose friends who share our interests, philosophy and background, we won't always see eye to eye. That's part of the pleasure of life, challenging us to open and develop maturity. Cutting off the possibility of viewing things from the other's point of view is cutting off our ability to view our world with an ever-broadening perspective.

How to Put It Right—
Dealing with Conflict in Friendship

Friends encourage and support each other in difficult times and generally make a positive impact on each other's lives. However, they're also willing to confront and constructively criticize and refuse to collude with what may lead to the eventual downfall of both the friend and the relationship. So let's take a look at how you can deal with conflict and with saying those things that your friend might not want to hear.

First of all, have a look at your motives for confronting the issue. Is your intention to communicate lovingly or is there part of you that wants to get your own back and hurt or put your friend down? If it's the latter then perhaps you need to take time to think, meditate and look at what the issue really is. In confronting whatever is going on between you, even if you're angry, you really need to be able to come from a position of openness and love if you're going to succeed in healing the wound and preserving the friendship.

So, in practical terms, take some time to get yourself grounded. Close your eyes for a moment and focus on your breathing. Then allow your heart chakra to open and send love to your friend while asking for insight about the problem and also that there will be the best possible outcome for both of you. This will enable you to be calm and open: to think and act rather than reacting and speaking in haste.

Try to clarify in your own mind and heart what the problem really is. By now you may have thought so much that more thinking will not get you very far. So just give yourself a few moments to allow any insight to simply drop into your mind. You may find yourself seeing things from a completely different perspective. When you feel clear, decide whether this is the time for you to confront your friend. Try to look at this from both points of view. It's important not to let things fester, let misunderstandings develop or avoid dealing with it, but there are instances when it's better to hold on for a while and choose the time and place carefully. For instance if your friend is already overwhelmed by stress, this might not be the time to add to it and expect a loving resolution. Similarly if you can't speak to her privately, wait till you can rather than embarrassing her in front of friends or family. Look also at your own needs. Are you calm enough to deal with the issue? Are you ready to deal with whatever she may have to say on the situation and about your behavior?

When you're ready, try to see the behavior you're upset about as completely separate from your friend. It's the behavior that you don't like, not your friend. Make sure that your verbal and non-verbal communication match each other. If your words say one thing while your body, your poise and your expression say another, there'll simply be more confusion for you both. With an attitude of concern for your mutual well-being, open with a statement that will help put you both at ease. Starting with "I" is generally least threatening and gets away from any feeling of accusation. For instance rather than "You never want to go where I want," you could say "I would like it if we took turns in choosing. . . ." Or "You're always putting me down" could become, "I'd like it if you saw me more as your equal."

If things get heated then try to suggest taking a breather and starting again. Your friend has just as much right to be assertive as you do and you may not like the things she has to say. But if you really mean to resolve the issue then you'll be open to her point of view. You own this friendship jointly and you're equal partners in it, or else it isn't a friendship at all. There's no need for you to do more of the work than she does on repairing it and looking after it, and if that's how it feels then perhaps you need to look at whether it really is a friendship or something that drags along for some underlying reason that you're not quite clear about. And remember that just as you took time to think before bringing up the issue, she might like to take time to think and come back to you with her new insights. Expecting that things will be resolved today just because *you're* ready to do so isn't really very loving. So if you have to wait awhile and have a second, or even third, conversation to try to resolve, accommodate or compromise, be patient. If you love each other the wait will be worth it.

What if it can't be resolved? Well, then you need to think whether you can accept your friend and the friendship even though there's something that irritates you. None of us is perfect, and that includes both you and your friend. In the words of a Turkish proverb, "Who seeks a faultless friend remains friendless." As with all relationships, it's the differences between us that challenge us to grow, enrich us and bring us more insight into who we really are. If your friendship doesn't allow for exploration of difficulties and is so fragile you don't dare approach conflict, then whether it is a loving friendship must be questioned. Friends mirror parts of us of which we may be unaware and some of which we may not like. In doing so they help us live out our truth, and show us we're lovable and acceptable even with all our faults and shortcomings.

Friends in Need . . .

There's a lovely old saying about stopping worrying about your own halo and starting to polish your friend's. When necessary, we must put ourselves aside for a while and let our love show in action by doing what the other needs: sometimes without being asked—just intuiting what's necessary.

In October 1998, there was severe flooding in Texas, 17 inches of rain falling in a 24-hour period. Apart from some minor flooding that didn't reach the house, I was spared. Many of the people whose homes lined the rivers were not so lucky. The great Colorado River, a mighty giant usually sleepily meandering its way to the ocean, became six miles wide in places and the Guadalupe, pale turquoise and silent, mesmerizing in its beauty, had, in one place at least, risen almost 50 feet to flood the area at each side of the ravine through which it flows. No one had expected that the water would ever reach that high, but the flood hit like a tidal wave, destroying everything in its path. Many homes were completely lost with all their contents; people were injured and there was some loss of life.

In 1999, I had the opportunity to talk to many of the survivors. Out of the disaster came stories of incredible heroic deeds—love in action: like the rancher who had taken his boat through turbulent waters now at treetop height, risking his life to rescue children stranded asleep and unaware in the care of a babysitter while their parents were washed ever further down the river from the home of neighbors they'd been visiting. Over the following weeks, neighbors had brought what they could share, had pitched in, hosing down carpets, retrieving furniture from downstream, digging out mud, finding lost animals and pets often still alive in the tops of trees. Some brought fresh water and ice, others food or clean linen. The whole community sprang into action, leaving clothing, food and household goods at churches, and rapidly set up emergency stations, all sharing from their hearts in the face of disaster. No one needed to be asked. People simply came from miles around and, as in the days of the frontiersmen and women, gave their friendship and love, suspending their own needs and their own lives for awhile to help restore the homes and dignity of their neighbors.

This is the love of friendship that is from the heart and the crown. It encompasses those we had never met, simply because they are human beings or living things and fellow inhabitants of the universe.

However, there is a time to do and a time to just stand there and be, offering our love as a witness as others find their way through disaster and back onto their feet—that's love in action too. Sometimes

Defeating loneliness

Perhaps the best cure for loneliness is to befriend someone, whether a person who is alone, elderly, sick, in prison, or even a child. Taking along a small gift in friendship makes you the recipient as well as the giver. Baking a cake for someone living alone will give you as much joy as it will give them. Even a smile or a kind word will help heal your wounds and change your life as well as that of the other person. Though there's healing in solitude that is chosen, loneliness is painful and demoralizing. Try to get out at least part of the day, or if you can't get out, talk to people on the phone. How about sitting down with your date book and making some social events well ahead of time so you always have something to look forward to? They don't have to be expensive treats—walking someone's dog in the park could be good for you and good for them. What about having a pet of your own, while being clear in your mind that it won't be a substitute for human relationships? Offering to babysit for a friend will do a good turn for you both. What about offering time at the local thrift shop? Being a volunteer in another way? Getting involved in some kind of service?

The more we involve ourselves in the service of others, the more our horizons widen, the more lovely people we meet, the more friends we make and the more our lives are transformed.

just standing there is harder than helping. I think that when I watch my mother struggle to pull herself up in the bed, her arthritic hands groping for the pulley, but knowing that every time she can do it for herself she'll have a feeling of accomplishment and it will keep her strong that much longer. It's not lack of care, but love, that makes me just stand there. The skill is in intuiting enough to get the balance right and feel when we need to move in to help.

No Longer Lovers but Friends

More than once I've heard couples say that really they should just have remained friends. Well, it obviously wasn't meant to be that way. But what is quite beautiful is if platonic friendship can remain after the phase of being lovers is over.

My ex-husband is my oldest friend. He has supported me through all the phases of my life since we met when I was 16. After a marriage spanning over two decades we've had a deep friendship for almost two decades more and the love between us has sustained us on a soul level though each of us has fallen in love again and committed to new relationships. I have no doubt that we'll go on supporting each other forever.

That ability to recognize the depth of friendship beyond the sexual intimacy that once marked the relationship is a mark of how people have loved each other. They can part and yet have concern for each other's highest good, letting go of whatever pain led to the parting. Truly loving in the first place—wanting the best for the other, whether or not that includes us—allows us the freedom of parting while we can hold onto the love. Particularly where there are children stuck in the middle of a crumbling relationship, it's wise to try to keep some communication open so that friendship can blossom again after the pain of separation is over. I know that where there is acrimony this can be a lofty ideal, but with forgiveness and an acknowledgment of the pact that brought us together in this lifetime (see page 202) we can release ourselves from one phase of intimacy and move into deep and sustaining friendship.

His, Hers and Our Friends

Sometimes when we move into a couple relationship, or get married, friends get lost along the way. We'll talk about that phase of falling in love and wanting only each other in the next chapter, and most good friends, while they may not like being sidelined will understand and give each other space. And of course the first priority should be the partnership, which embodies a friendship that no other can replicate. But a strong partnership allows space for other people too who can, as friends, enrich and bring freshness to the couple relationship.

Sometimes problems arise when one forgets that in general men and women see friendship differently. Men often have several casual friends to whom they're attracted by a sharing of concepts and activities, with whom they joke and banter, while avoiding deep personal communication. Others have deep, respectful and reserved friendships which span years during which little of a personal nature is ever exchanged despite the fact that there is a profound bond. Two women often base their friendship on feeling, developing deep close friendships with a lot of verbal exchange, as they share their thoughts, hopes and fears along with confidences that they feel only another woman would understand. Such friendships may appear frivolous, yet they are sustaining and profoundly supportive, relieving much of the pressure that would otherwise fall on the partnership. This tendency to keep some friends separately is often healthy though care needs to be taken to protect time for the prime partnership.

Many couples opt more for friendships that involve them both, usually with other couples, finding their circle of friends enriched as single friends take partners who then become part of the group. Some feel more comfortable with these joint friends since the likelihood is that they will meet together and therefore time with friends is not time apart.

Platonic Friendship

It's been said that platonic friendships—that is, close friendships without a sexual element—cannot exist between men and women. That is not so. Though the similarities between two men or two women may lay a better foundation for friendship, a man and a woman may share similar desires and inclinations and complement each other so well that true friendship, lifting them beyond sexuality to a place of spiritual communion, becomes possible. The same benevolent love that is often the hallmark of same-sex friendship, in which each gives to the other to render them more complete, may even be superseded in platonic friendship since each person, coming from a different sexual stance, has a broader experience to offer the other. In such a relationship the woman often leads the man to learn more of his deep emotional self, his intuition and feelings, while she may learn from him a new clarity of thought, power and strength. Though the ideal is to find all of those within the inner marriage of masculine and feminine (see page 204), platonic friendships can help lead us to that realization of our wholeness and be an enriching experience. Personal communion rather than sexual attraction is the overriding essence. This mutual love, which helps us complete ourselves and the other, is often the basis of platonic friendship.

Affirmation

I open my heart today to approach those I meet in loving friendship and remain open to receive their love also. Wherever necessary, let forgiveness bring freedom.

Meditation

Take yourself to your safe place and make sure that you have sufficient time and that you will be comfortable and won't be disturbed.

Now, close your eyes and focus on your breathing. Relax and let go of any anxiety. Breathe in the white light that surrounds you. Know that you are protected.

Focus on your heart chakra and feel the warm glow of love as it starts to open now. Let that loving feeling spread throughout your body and out into your aura, cleansing, healing, balancing every part of you. Feel a sense of peace and serenity surrounding you.

With a single breath, imagine yourself surrounded by friends. Some of these may be people you already know. Others may not yet have made themselves known to you. Send each one love from your heart to theirs. Slowly look around you and as you do be acutely aware of all of the good things that these friends are bringing into your life. Take a few minutes and make a mental list of their good qualities. Look at them with love, understanding and compassion. You know that like you they have their faults, but they have more abundant good characteristics. As you appreciate each and every one of them, smile inwardly at each of them and thank them for being in your life, for the things they are teaching you, for the things you've already shared and still have to share. See them within the beam of divine light that surrounds you all and flow love into the relationship that exists or will exist between you.

In this moment, while remaining grounded, shine your own divine light into the heart of each one, and feel their love for you. Give each a message if you wish, or give a message to the whole assembly of friends there in front of you and be still and listen for anything that might come to you from them.

Hold your friends in love for as long as you wish and when you're ready just allow them to fade gently from your view. Let all the love from them enter your heart before you allow it to close to the point where it feels most comfortable.

Now start once again to be aware of your breathing. Feel your physical presence. Move your fingers and toes and start to return now to a place behind your eyes. Make sure that you're grounded. Take it easy, and when you're ready gently open your eyes and be fully present. Stretch a little and have a drink of water before you record in your journal anything you wish.

Eight

The Perfect Mate

I love thee freely as men strive for Right;
I love thee purely, as they turn from Praise.
I love thee with the passion put to use
In my old griefs, and with my childhood's faith.
I love thee with a love I seemed to lose
With my lost saints!—I love thee with the breath,
Smiles, tears, of all my life!—and, if God choose,
I shall but love thee better after death.

—ELIZABETH BARRETT BROWNING,
"SONNETS FROM THE PORTUGUESE," XLIII

Though I've titled this chapter "The Perfect Mate," many may ask, "Does such a thing exist?" For many, romantic relationships are a minefield and what starts off as the perfect fairytale partnership often ends up in tears and acrimony, both parties feeling sad and disillusioned, cynical about whether *love* exists, let alone a perfect mate. But true romantic love does exist, and when you experience it, it can completely transform you. And as for the perfect mate—well, read on.

This chapter aims to help you better understand loving partnerships, your reaction to them and why you may repeat patterns that lead you into pain, or why so far you've felt unsuccessful in love. If you're in a wonderful relationship then I'm happy for you. But you may still find something that can be improved for the two of you. A word of caution: please don't expect to find something here that you can use to change your partner to make the relationship work. The only person you can change is you, but I assure you that if you do that, your relationship will change.

Your relationship is your business and no one else's; so is your choice of partner and your sexual orientation. No one has a perfect formula that works for everyone. No one knows how you feel about your partner. And I can only share what I believe, have experienced or observed. What's right for me might not be so for you or anyone else, and that's okay! If it feels good and right for you, enjoy it. Feel with your heart; intuit where you are, and don't let anyone rain on your parade or lead you to be dissatisfied. Dissecting why you feel the way you do may not be what you need to do. Let what you read here merely enhance it.

But if your relationship feels disappointing, wrong or painful and if you've been in this place before, then perhaps you've been called to read this so you can start to make changes. Be gentle with yourself and your partner if you have one, and sleep on any changes you suddenly feel you want to make. If they're right, they'll still feel like a good idea tomorrow. If you need to, talk things over with someone. But mainly, trust yourself.

Can Romantic Love Last Forever?

So much has been written about romantic love, and yet most would agree that it's not the romantic phase that endures, but more what M. Scott Peck has termed the superglue of love—that which binds us even in the hard times and holds us together even when we're fed up and would like to run away. It's what brings us home even when someone attractive may come on to us at a party; that touches our heart when we wake in the morning and the person next to us has messed-up hair and swollen, sleepy eyes and we think they look beautiful. It's what makes a couple together for 40 years still walk arm in arm down the street and kiss each other when they leave the house or return.

So does romantic love really exist or is it simply a construct of our culture? If for awhile we can be so in love that it feels as though we've glimpsed the face of God, how is it that sometimes, after only a brief while, the feelings are gone and we wonder what it was that attracted us so? A trick of the light, some hormonal aberration, a chemical reaction, a glitch in our consciousness or even an apparent loss of consciousness altogether?! Or could it be that for awhile, no matter how brief, the object of our affection *did* fit perfectly what we needed? That perhaps they reflected something for us, prompted some constellation of events that gave us a peek at what, otherwise, we might not have seen?

Falling in Love and Loving

If you've fallen head over heels in love, it's an experience you'll never forget. Indeed I had one lady in her fifties who came along to see me worrying about the fading of her undoubted beauty. She'd never been in a long relationship but had had many brief liaisons. She loved being in love, but as soon as the heady feelings started to fade she'd opt out before a relationship could develop, and would search again for a new face to give her the high she sought. It was the romance that was her turn-on, but the thought of responsibility and commitment to a proper relationship she found frightening.

Oh that the in-love phase could last for ever! So I sometimes hear people lament. But how exhausting that would be. All that adrenaline rush as we wait with fast-beating heart and panting breath for a mere sight of the beloved, unable to sleep or eat. Being permanently in love would screw up the rest of your life!

When we fall in love, for awhile we forget who we are, our individual boundaries falling as we rush into each other's space, aura mingling with aura, chakras bonding; we become a single unit that cannot contemplate separation for an instant. Do you remember that? We just can't get enough of each other. This in-loveness has been called the purest form of insanity, and certainly in that state we often find ourselves doing things that we otherwise wouldn't do.

But the state of loving is a more comfortable and companionable state, with a sense of deep enduring devotion, affection, care, trust, support and respect. Our boundaries are back in place, and we have no illusions about who we are individually and who we are as a couple. The strong boundary around us both tells the world that we're an item. We know that we can be angry with each other and not fall apart; spend time apart and still be together; disagree but accommodate our differences; protect each other fiercely if necessary and be secure in the knowledge that we're there for each other. We'll still have ups and downs, but the relationship is stable.

The really lucky ones have learned the knack of falling in love with each other repeatedly. Having found the gentle contentment of loving each other, every now and then a special event awakens all the old magic and they fall in love again. Back in the normal routine of life, they happily return to loving and getting on with their ordinary day. This, I believe, is the pinnacle of coupleship and the hallmark of the good and lasting relationship.

For some, letting go of the in-love phase is laced with disappointment. They think the fairytale's over. But in fact it's where the fairytale begins.

Our lives, and loves, go in cycles. And if we look at relationships there are cycles there too, with good times, fallow times, in-between times and bad times. Sometimes as the cycle turns and we have a bad time, we decide to leave, whereas others fight through it and as the cycle turns find themselves more closely bound by mutual suffering with renewed strength and happiness. Sometimes it's only the memory of the good times, even though they may be fleeting and far between, that keeps people clinging when there's more bad than good.

Why We Choose Whom We Choose

There were times when people made choices of partner for us on the basis of family and social background, financial security and power. In some cultures that's still the case. I've spoken to couples whose marriage was arranged and who've grown to respect and love each other deeply, though whether they ever went through the phase of falling in love is another matter. Some say they're grateful that a choice was made for them because otherwise they would have let their hearts rule their heads and made choices that might not have led to the solid foundation they've found. There are others who for the rest of their lives have harbored feelings of love for someone who was deemed unsuitable for them, and many who have felt exploited, hardly consulted and who endure a life of misery.

Left to our own devices, our choice is guided by a multitude of factors, many of which are unconscious: temperament, our individual makeup, our past relationships with family members and others, our sexual orientation, our social and intellectual background, religion, race, interests, inner sexual balance and of course sexual attraction, to name but a few. Though you might think that opposites attract, it's the things that are similar that really bring us together. We tend to choose a partner who matches us along several parameters—someone who in some way is like us.

It's a truism that the things that attract us in the first place can be the things that eventually drive us apart. Whatever causes us to choose a partner, we'd be wise to choose carefully, for as the eleventh-century French theologian, St. Bernard of Clairvaux pointed out, "That which we love we come to resemble." In a real sense, we often become more and more like those with whom we identify and share love.

Similarities That Bring Us Together

Sometimes at the beginning of a workshop, I ask everyone to wander around for awhile then choose someone to sit next to without speaking to each other at all. After a few minutes almost everyone will pair off. I then ask them to talk to each other about their backgrounds, and they're often amazed to find that, without a word having been spoken, they've chosen someone with a quite marked similarity. Perhaps it is that there was addiction or violence in the family; that they've been pushed to do well and even overachieve; that family problems were never discussed at all; that they're now middle class but came from a lower-class background; that they came from immigrant families, that they have a similar religious background, etc. In one workshop everyone was amused when out of 36 people two doctors, two opera singers, two senior executives (each the younger brother in a poor family), two elder sisters who had problems with relationships, and two children of families that had been involved in a tragedy where a family member had been killed found each other—all without the benefit of a single verbal clue. What's more, they found that those who had suffered tragedies had done so at around the same age. The only people who couldn't seem to find anyone and eventually just sat down together but couldn't really talk to each other had been abandoned children, fostered or adopted, and had never had a sense of belonging anywhere.

The signals we pick up are from information displayed in nonverbal behavior such as gestures and posture, but more specifically, energy carried in our aura. As we discussed in Chapter 2, our aura meets people before we do and, before we utter a word, a massive amount of information is exchanged. Let's imagine that someone lost a parent at the age of six when the sacral chakra was just developing. The damage to that chakra and the pattern of resultant difficulty in development of those chakras above it will be similar to that of someone else who suffered a similar loss at a similar age and the two sacral chakras recognize that long before the two people ever discuss it with each other. Two people may come together with seemingly little in common, only to find out later that they both had fathers who were unpredictable and tended to shout and threaten. Though the problem may show up later as a power struggle, their solar plexuses knew this from the beginning and are helping each other to sort out the issue!

Sometimes there are negative repercussions. Imagine two people coming together who, as children, had to take care of a sick parent. What happens when each of them wants to be the caretaker of the other? Or if each had a mother who was cold and unloving—where will they have learned to nourish and care for each other? Later we'll look at how this can lead to separation and repeating the pattern unless we sort it out now.

What's important is that once we become aware of why we keep choosing the same kind of person, the fatal attraction they have for us, and we for them, subsides and we can choose someone more suited to who we are now.

Masculine–Feminine Balance

Our inner balance of the masculine and feminine is governed initially by the sacral chakra, but every chakra makes its contribution to enable us to perform in harmony like a talented orchestra.

The inner masculine part of us, the masculine principle, is governed by the left brain and deals with such functions as organizational skills, action, ambition, drive, protection, providing and logic. The inner feminine principle is governed by the right side of your brain and deals with verbal skills, creativity, music, art, nurturing, mothering, holding and other soft and less-structured gifts. Ideally, as we develop, we learn to use all of our gifts in balance, giving us a broad field of skills that enable us to be independent, flexible, healthy adults.

But if for some reason we don't have an inner balance, then we're likely to choose someone else who isn't very balanced either, and who has the things that we don't have. So a very feminine woman who hasn't developed her masculine principle will be more likely to fall for a very masculine man who will have what she lacks. Two people with a strong inner masculine who come together generally lock horns regularly and have difficulties with aggression in the relationship, whereas two people with a strong inner feminine coming together have some difficulty in organization and in leading the relationship down a path in life. Where people are balanced within themselves, they tend to look for someone else who is similarly balanced.

This balancing of the masculine and feminine both individually and within the couple applies to any combination of the sexes. The inner marriage of the two principles allows for partnership between those of the same sex to be similarly perfected in love. The ideal situation is to be able to merge in a partnership with another while keeping our own individuality.

Eventually of course we can get to the point where we don't need any skills from anyone else to balance us, and then we choose to get together from a place of want rather than need.

"Unequal" Partnerships

Some partnerships appear unequal, and it's difficult to see where the similarities are that brought the two parties together. They may be from very different backgrounds, of widely differing ages, opposite social environments and intellects. Occasionally such relationships last for a long time and are deeply satisfying for both parties, though more often they burn fiercely for a while then peter out and die. Though they may seem to be born of lack of judgement or poor choice, usually something much more profound is at work and each party is gaining something. Not only are there past-life issues to consider (see Appendix 2) but sometimes one soul has contracted to heal a less-evolved one, bringing it to a more courageous and honorable way of living in the light.

Such seemingly unequal relationships occur when one person exerts external power while the other has authentic, inner power. What appears to be resignation and submission of the one is in fact their unwillingness to move from a position of individual empowerment into competition with the other. Occasionally the true power balance is revealed only in times of crisis.

> Tammy and Jack were an unusual couple. Tammy appeared timid and quiet, and Jack's family often wondered what on earth he'd seen in this unassuming, plain girl when he could have had his pick of the attractive young women who swarmed around the young rugby player. At family gatherings she seemed withdrawn and everyone had doubts when Jack announced their engagement. Over the years Tammy kept a low profile and appeared not to change while Jack continued up the corporate ladder, becoming more and more successful. Jack's parents were very proud of him, and from time to time discussed their concern about the fact that he needed a more supportive wife who would be more at ease with the business world he now inhabited.
>
> But what they didn't see was what Jack really had. Underneath his sometimes tough, abrasive exterior, his

quick wit and his dazzling smile, Jack was vulnerable and fragile, his mood often brittle and his self-confidence poor. Tammy, on the other hand, was filled with quiet wisdom and self-esteem that led her to be self-contained and calm, which had often been mistaken by Jack's family as her being withdrawn and stand-offish. With a touch and a smile she could soothe Jack. With a word she could breathe power into him that could get him through the toughest negotiation. And with her, he was soft and gentle and at home in a way that he'd never felt with another human being. The true power balance in the relationship could have been in Tammy's favor except that her love for him was such that she wanted only his empowerment and his freedom, his well-being and his happiness, for she already had all those things for herself.

The truth of the relationship only became apparent to Jack's family when he was unconscious following a car crash. In the hospital where his parents were rushing round doing things and pestering the nurses about taking care of their boy, Tammy simply sat and held his hand, occasionally brushed his cheek with her fingers and whispered to him. The few words she uttered to medical and nursing staff held an authority they hadn't witnessed before, and she expressed praise and gratitude for all that was being done for her husband. The air of peace around the couple became almost visible as for the first time, Tammy allowed Jack's parents to see where the real power lay: within her and her amazingly powerful love for their son. Tammy, for her part, gained much from Jack's extrovert display, which opened doors for her she would otherwise not have known existed.

Temporary chaos in relationships

Though it's good to have peace in our relationships, sometimes you may need the spice of a little drama or chaos to shake you up and get your attention. For it's in times of crisis that the seeds of new order are sown. So don't worry if you're going through a particularly argumentative phase in your relationship.

Chaos can make you take a fresh look at what you really want and what's of real value to who you truly are. It allows you to recommit to your life's purpose, to reassess your path and those with whom you choose to tread it. Sometimes it indicates that for a time you need to be alone if you are to follow your divine path and prevent your message from getting lost in a morass of human feelings.

We might like to blame our partners for the pain we find ourselves suffering, but actually there is both mutual benefit and growth and they deserve our gratitude, understanding and compassion, for often we're the catalysts in each other's spiritual growth or catapult each other's return to our rightful path.

As the fabric of our lives is tattered by chaos, we're forced to make choices we'd otherwise avoid. Sometimes we have remained in pain for years, then one day, almost inexplicably, a shift occurs and we free ourselves. We can only assume at that point the experience was complete and there was no longer a need to stay.

Learning to keep working on ourselves, one step ahead of the game, often allows us a relatively painless ascent, though the challenges in life will always prompt growth and creativity, forcing us to shed all that no longer fits and don the mantle of our new life.

Authentic inner power always demonstrates itself by empowering the other; by encouraging growth, independence and true learning. It's only those who are uncertain of their true power who need to wield it over others, and they do so by exerting control, rescuing and rendering others helpless.

Does any of this ring true for you? It's important that you remember who you are. If you're in any doubt, go back to Chapter 4, on loving yourself. You have amazing qualities and are a very powerful being. But you must have the courage to use this power wisely. Whatever brought the two of you together into an unusual relationship is no one's business but yours. Similarly what keeps you there, only you really know. Such apparently unequal partnerships demand courage from both of you, since sadly there will often be someone who will refuse to accept your choice. That's okay. It's not their relationship. But if in honesty you know there are less than honorable reasons for you to be together, though you must still learn from the relationship and so must your partner, perhaps you need to look at how you're going to extricate yourself with the least possible harm to you both.

Finding Your Soul Mate

Have you felt that all-encompassing love that you just know has been there always and will go on forever more? That you *know* this person even though you've just met? This is the great love of Dante and Beatrice; the love of Solomon in the Song of Songs. The passion that we feel lucky to have found in a lifetime even if life dictates that somehow we're separated. This feeling of having always known each other—that's the meeting with your soul mate, the wonder and delight of which changes our lives forever.

So is there only one soul mate for us? Well, no. Though sadly some are destined never to find one, it is possible to reconnect with more than one soul mate in a lifetime.

We'll talk about this more in Appendix 2, but briefly, we've lived out diverse roles in numerous lifetimes and are meeting again to complete old promised tasks. Sometimes the meeting is full of knowing from the first moment, what we call love at first sight, though sometimes it develops over time.

A beautiful spiritual woman I met was about to be married. She told me they'd met by chance (if such a thing exists!) almost 16 years earlier, only days after her husband-to-be had become engaged. In that second she recognized him as her soul mate. However, he married and she saw no more of him until 11 years later when they met again in exactly the same place. He'd been divorced for four years and she for eight. Instantly they recognized each other and fell in love. She said that in so many ways they simply *knew* each other. Both had worked out various issues in marriages with other people and were now free to be together.

Many people have a sense of knowing each other from another time. For some the evidence is even more astounding. Often soul mate relationships are fascinating and filled with delight, peaceful and calm and always harmonious. However, being with a soul mate sometimes isn't that way. Often they press our buttons in a way that no one else can. They separate us from our fragile state of peace so that we can grow. In fact they're our most loving teachers. Underlying their actions is a profound love that understands and is willing to challenge us. We may have been doing the same thing with each other for centuries. Finding a soul mate doesn't necessarily mean that we'll always be with them, though we may, till death do us part.

For if we reach the point where we've experienced together all we contracted to do in this lifetime, we'll part, possibly to come together again in another life. We've fulfilled our promises for now and we can love each other enough to let go. It's often in the letting go with love and with a genuine desire for the other's welfare that we see the sign of the true soul mate. The film *Step Mom* (1999) shows beau-

---

Finding a soul mate or falling madly in love?

With a soul mate there is:

- *a sense of having known them before, or even forever*
- *instant familiarity*
- *a feeling of being spiritual partners, of there being something between you that transcends "humanness"*
- *a sense of belonging from the instant you meet, rather than just compatibility*
- *instant love rather than love that develops over time*
- *a sense that the love includes all humanity*
- *inspiration and energy*
- *a feeling that there are no barriers between you*
- *the sense of being partners*
- *the fact that (sometimes) you have similar facial features*
- *a sharing of similar spiritual (not necessarily religious) values*
- *a feeling of a shared mission or purpose*
- *a feeling of being constantly together even if you're miles apart*

---

tifully the possible sequence of pairing with soul mates. The love of the original couple who have parted while still caring deeply for each other isn't invalidated by the presence of a new soul mate partnership.

Accepting Each Other as You Are

Acceptance is a two-way street. It's easy to forget that, while we're struggling to accept things we're irritated by, we have habits that our partners are having difficulty accepting too. In fact the things that threaten and challenge us are those that are prompting us to learn to accommodate and compromise. Our lovers test our tolerance and push us to broaden the range of what we can accept with equanimity. If we feel pained and disturbed it's because part of us hasn't stretched enough to accept. But you might ask, why should we? The answer is

---

Rage and hatred

If you're at the point where resentment has become rage, and love has turned to hatred, then your underlying fear needs to be explored. Often this is something deep and of the past—perhaps even of another lifetime—and you're being challenged to heal it. It's indifference rather than hatred that really spells the ending of a relationship.

---

that that's what growth is all about. That's why we're with them in the first place.

Learning to broaden your tolerance is one thing, but if there are many issues that pain you, perhaps you should look at why you're still in the situation. Where your integrity or your heartfelt principles and desires are constantly challenged, it's time to sort out what the message really is here. Are you being asked to look at and possibly change your stance, or to have the courage to stand up for what you hold dear and move on? Is part of the learning for your partner that they cannot behave in this way and expect someone to remain with them? Spend a little time searching your heart and asking to be shown the answer. It might come to you in the most unexpected way.

I Can Only Change Me

As I said earlier, I can only change me. But how often have you heard someone say (or even thought yourself), "Oh, he'll change!" Within that statement is the seed of trouble, for it means that only when the other person has altered, are they truly acceptable to us. It usually also indicates that we think we'll be able to effect that change. Sometimes the extent to which one person wants the other to change is astounding and I wonder why they ever thought they matched in the first place.

And then there's perfectionism!

A lovely young woman came to see me in tears. She was
deeply loved by her husband of four years, but she said
that she'd already changed so much to try to accommodate
him that she'd started to feel as though she no longer
existed as the person she was. We decided that the three of
us should meet and I hoped that he would confirm his love
for her, and that her fears that she couldn't match up to
what he wanted in a wife would be unfounded. However,
though he did profess his love for her very eloquently, and
complimented her for some of her attributes, he then
launched into a list of ways in which she was not perfect
and where he would like her to change to please him. I
referred him to the following story:

A woman was walking by a dress shop one day and
saw a beautiful pink dress in the window. It had long
flowing sleeves, a draped neckline and a swinging skirt that
would fall almost to her ankles. It was decorated with tiny
pearl beads and the chiffon set off their beauty. She was so
taken with the beautiful garment that she immediately
went into the shop to buy it.

She tried it on and the sales lady complimented her
on how the dress enhanced her figure and how well she
suited the color. The woman looked at herself in the
mirror and twirled around.

"Yes, I'll have it," she said. "But I'd like the hem
shortened and the sleeves only elbow length. Perhaps
instead of the little pearl beads I could have shell buttons
and we could do away with the zip at the back. I think the
skirt would be better if we lose some of this material. I'd
like it a little more straight. And do you have it in blue?"

The sales lady smiled at her wisely.

"Madam," she said, "I think you ought to buy a different dress."

How ludicrous that story sounds. We would rarely expect such an array of alterations in a garment we were buying. And yet often I see couples expecting so many changes in each other. And though it's natural that couples change as they come together, if we get into a relationship expecting that we'll change the other, then we're generally in for a shock.

Loving communication is everything! The two of you need to talk about the things you find difficult to accept about each other, though this must be done in a spirit of love—and a bit of humor wouldn't go amiss! To say to your partner with an arm around their shoulder that you'd like to explore together some way to keep the house tidier is rather different from exclaiming that you don't know how your partner can live in this mess. How about suggesting that there could be a place where you can be ultra tidy and she can be as messy as she likes, but that the rest of the house is homely and lived in but not littered? How about some humorous signal that her mess is encroaching on your space and you'd like it to stop multiplying by the minute? How about offering a joint tidying session before the new demarcation line is drawn? How about deciding that you'll think and act rather than reacting? Not always easy, but worth cultivating. What about looking at the fact that it might be you who needs to change? Have you been willing to come halfway?

But there are times when you just know that you can change no further, and that accommodating any more threatens your integrity. When what you're being asked to accept is simply unacceptable. What then? Well, though you need to remain committed to being present and open to opportunities to grow (and there are certainly challenges being thrown at you that are prompting growth!) you have to decide what's best for *you*. Honor yourself. If you can remain loving, under-standing and compassionate, staying within your own space, holding onto your own standards, morals and integrity in the face of disap-pointments and shattered expectations and not resort to retaliation and revenge, then that's fine. But if the answer is that you cannot, then perhaps you need to accept that it's time to take care of your-self and separate from what is giving you such pain. We'll look at leaving later.

Meeting Each Other's Needs and Desires

When we were little girls, my sister and I were taught to gratefully receive whatever we were given and not to ask for anything else. The intention was quite beautiful, but it's been a hard lesson for me to let go of, and sometimes I still struggle with it, finding it hard to ask for my needs to be fulfilled, but then sometimes feeling dissatisfied and disappointed when they aren't. Expecting that others can read our minds (even though in the first flush of love it appears they can) is both unfair and foolish.

As a child I longed to play the piano and finally had lessons, though we didn't have a piano at home. My grandparents said that I could practice at their house not far away. It wasn't a happy experi-ence. As loving as my grandparents were, sometimes it just wasn't convenient for me to practice. Though I loved the music, it eventu-ally became torture to go there to practice and I gave up my lessons. In my twenties, I casually mentioned in conversation that I'd always wanted a piano of my own. I was delightfully shocked when on my next birthday, a somewhat old and battered but nevertheless quite serviceable piano appeared in the living room. I could hardly leave it alone for weeks. It amazed me that one of my desires had been real-ized so apparently effortlessly. My husband, happy and simultane-ously amused at my joyous reaction, asked what else I'd been silently

Feeding each other's desires

A man died and arrived at the gates of heaven. He was met there by the gatekeeper who had a huge ledger in which were noted all the deeds of the man's life. The gatekeeper scratched his head.

"You're a very unusual case," he said. "You have exactly the same number of good deeds as bad deeds and so you can choose whether you're to go to heaven or hell."

The man thought for a moment, and then decided that he would have a look at hell since it might be a bit more fun than heaven. He was duly dispatched and arrived in hell to find a huge banqueting hall with tables laid with exquisite glass and silver, damask cloths and sumptuous food. Around the table there were people dressed in fine evening wear, but they all looked very sad. He then noticed each person had a spoon attached to each arm, the handle being so long that it was impossible to reach their mouths with the food.

The man looked at the misery on the faces of the people there and decided he would prefer to be in heaven. On arriving there, however, he was shocked initially to find that there were identical tables laid with similar finery, and the people sitting there had similar spoons attached to their arms. The difference was they were smiling and happy. When he looked around, he saw why. Though they could not reach their own mouths, each was feeding someone else with the food of their choice.

The gatekeeper smiled as the reality dawned upon the man.

"Make sure you keep it heavenly," he said. "You could soon make this hell if someone wants one thing and instead you put something else into their mouth."

longing for, and suddenly a new world opened up in which, quite gingerly at first, I began to name what I would like. It was great. But I still wonder if I would ever have asked had I not been so generously invited to do so.

So to a large extent, having your needs met is your own responsibility, and asking sensitively (not demanding!) is fine. This goes for all aspects of the relationship, including sex. It's perfectly okay to say what you like and what would please you. Your partner has the same right, of course! Sometimes, however, we need to think hard about what we feel comfortable giving, no matter what our partner wants.

What's painful is to make the other aware of your needs and to have these dismissed as unimportant. But in the real world there are times when we just have to learn to live with not getting what we want. Learning to be honest about what you need is a gift in communication. And when your partner asks for what he needs, it's kind to give him that rather than what you want for him, unless there's some particular reason why you shouldn't. Sometimes the desires of the other stretch our integrity and make us uncomfortable, and if this is so, it's better to be honest and say so rather than do something that hurts us and ultimately threatens the relationship.

One of my clients was in a difficult marriage with a man she truly loved but who was in chaos. She cried sadly in her session when reporting that her husband's birthday was approaching and she'd planned a present. However, he'd said that if she really loved him and wanted to please him she would buy him cocaine for his birthday so that he could have a binge!

Communication

I've been known to say that all relationship problems are issues of poor communication. In fact I might go further than that and say that all problems full stop are problems of communication. By communication, I don't just mean talking. Though casually chatting is fun, and talking on a superficial level is what we do much of the time, there are times that call for deep communication, which is a whole new state of being.

If you think you're really communicating with your partner, just stop a moment and check it out. Either bring to mind your chakra system or have another look at Chapter 2. Then run down the following checklist:

- Is your root chakra open so that you remain solidly grounded and strong, looking after your own survival above everything?

- Is your sacral chakra open to allow you to be flexible and open to the other person with a willingness to change?

- Is your solar plexus chakra reminding you of your own power but also that you must not use it to disempower anyone else?

- Is your heart chakra open with love and compassion and the ability to empathize with your partner? Have you checked on your motives so that your communication comes truly from your heart and not from your ego? Are you viewing your partner with respect, loyalty, appreciation and admiration, seeing her as someone of worth and beauty?

- Is your throat chakra open so that you can speak your truth and voice your integrity with gentleness and patience but with strength and clarity and also listen attentively without judgement or interruption? Do you have a genuine desire to share the best information you have?

- Is your brow open with the vision of what you really desire for you and the relationship?

- Are you open to a flow of divine love, which will bless you both and enable you to come to the best possible conclusion for you both?

- Is your whole being protected so that if there is anger and fear, you don't need to pick it up?

- Are you sure that your non-verbal signals match your verbal ones?

If you can answer yes honestly to all of the above and are satisfied with what you've found at each level, you're ready to communicate from a place of love rather than fear, concern rather than accusation, and a positive outcome is inevitable. That magic alchemy that promotes communication in its finest form is present and you are ready to show who you are and what you believe. This doesn't mean that you'll get what you want. It doesn't mean that you'll dazzle your partner with your articulate delivery and that they'll fall into your arms agreeing with everything you say. But it does mean that, whatever the outcome, you came from your soul and spoke your truth as you understand it in this moment. Tomorrow, you may feel different, and that's fine. You can update your communication again whenever you wish.

With no sacrifice of the unique individuality of either, and in perfect freedom, the lives of two people who communicate in this way seem to flow together, integrating till they appear to function harmoniously as a single unit. There's often a palpable magic around such couples who live in perfect accord, celebrating the divinity of each other and of all life. Each is self-aware with pure motives and, through the gracious application of respect, gentleness, understanding and love, calls into active expression the latent good in the other. Now this is something worth striving for!

Believing in Each Other, Learning from Each Other

If you can respect each other as equal teachers and students, with unique messages for each other, there's a basis for love laced with a good deal of gratitude, despite the fact that sometimes what's being passed between you may not feel very good and in some cases may be downright painful. Acknowledging that what you're both experiencing is developing your soul can soothe the most difficult of situations, and help you to let go of resistance and suck all the juice without too much pain.

In loving, and therefore wanting the highest possible good for the beloved, we automatically aim high. For as Desiré Joseph Mercier, the Belgian prelate and philosopher, said, "We must not only give what we have but give what we are." Our partner's spiritual growth becomes as important as our own. And as we consciously think and act in a compassionate, loving and healing way that facilitates the other's well-being, we ourselves automatically grow too and have more of ourselves to give. Thus in a truly spiritual partnership, in which each is committed to the other's highest good, there's constant change as we accommodate each other's insights and rejoice in them.

But if you have a codependent partnership that fails to acknowledge the spiritual element, though your feelings may be strong and both of you talk of love, with a verbal commitment to each other's welfare, petty jealousies, anger and resentments cause stasis, and growth ceases. Should one of you then struggle to continue to grow, the other is threatened with the underlying fear of abandonment, separation and loss overriding the possible joy at the other's achievements. In order to maintain the relationship, either the one must deny the desire to grow or the other must grow also. But since codependence usually exists against a background of damage, the fear often outweighs the joy and antagonism ensues, with increased chaos and drama. We'll be looking at this more later.

Conflict in Love

"If you would learn the secret of right relations look only for the good, that is the Divine, in everything and leave the rest to God." So said author J. Allen Boone. A wonderful theory and one that works if we're able to keep to it, but in practice few of us are able to con-

Dealing with conflict self-assertively

- Work with only one issue at a time—don't bring in the past, old arguments, etc., that confuse the situation and lead you to forget what you're really talking about.
- If things get too heated, take a break, with a commitment to reconvene in half an hour.
- Try talking on neutral ground where you'll be more likely to talk than shout.
- Use "I" statements that show that you're taking responsibility for your own part in the conflict rather than accusing the other.
- Try to see it from the other's point of view and don't gloat over the insights your partner may have—if he suddenly realizes he was wrong, accept that graciously and move on.
- Try to keep in mind the goal is to heal and not to wound.
- If criticism is necessary then make sure it's constructive and apt, not exaggerated and cruel. If you use words like "always" and "never," you're already out of order. (For example "You always have to have your own way," "You've never allowed me to. . . .")
- See yourselves as a team united against the problem. This will encourage you to find a solution to a situation that neither of you likes.
- Go into separate rooms and brainstorm possible solutions on a piece of paper. You might be surprised to find that you're both thinking along the same lines.
- Try to see the problem as divorced from the two of you. Psychologically set it to one side so that both of you can see it as an issue rather than a part of the other you don't like or want.
- If a solution can't be found to the whole problem, is there a step each of you can take towards the middle to accommodate the other in some small way? This can often be accepted as a token of good will and may diffuse the situation.

sistently carry out such a lofty ideal. And in any case, disagreement and conflict form a natural and essential part of relationships.

Sometimes I meet a couple who've been together for years and who say, "We've never had a cross word." Well, if that's so, I find it worrying!

A healthy relationship demands two healthy, whole individuals who are inwardly secure with good boundaries. They're held with gentleness and strength by bonds of love that are strong enough to withstand conflict. Confrontation, with a willingness to look at what creates insecurity and instability in the relationship, allows each to grow and the union to flourish. We become more conscious of the other's vulnerabilities as well as strengths and the desire to help each other heal deepens both the love and the commitment to the relationship. However, if conflict becomes more common than peace, there's a problem.

A mutually empowering solution to conflict can always be found if you both have a commitment to work as a team towards this. Standing on opposing sides simply leads to a situation where one of you can win but the other loses. In such cases, the relationship always loses too. Resolving to take a little time to walk in the other person's shoes can make things seem very different!

If you can trust that what you divulge will be handled with loving care and not hurled back at you during argument and feel safe to honestly express anger and fear, with the intention to heal rather than to wound, there should be a way to resolution. Remembering this isn't always easy in the heat of the moment. But approaching conflict with courage and self-assertion can yield a great harvest. Remember —your partner has a right to be self-assertive too.

Dealing with even long-standing conflict can be easier than you imagine as long as you set some rules for dealing with it assertively. But sometimes things have got to the point where simply trying to talk about what's going on isn't enough.

Elizabeth came along to see me complaining of a long-standing problem with her boyfriend, Sam, whom she loved and had lived with for about four years before parting because of recurrent arguments that were damaging them both. They were still committed to each other and saw each other most days when she would stop at his apartment close by on her way home from work. Often they would have a meal and spend some time together before she went home; however, despite making repeated resolutions to have a pleasant evening, they often ended up in the same old argument and would part feeling sad, painful, drained and confused as to why it had happened again.

Sam agreed to come to the next session. He was warm and affectionate and appeared to be committed to working to improve things.

First we looked for common ground. They both wanted to marry and Elizabeth wanted a commitment to have children. Sam wanted to reinstate their sex life though Elizabeth was a bit reluctant, feeling scared to allow herself to be vulnerable. Elizabeth wanted Sam to contribute more to the finances. Though he was very generous with his time and affection and was willing to share chores, she felt that he could earn more if he extended himself; then she'd have to shoulder less of the financial burden. Sam wanted time to write and pursue his creative talents, though that meant that he'd opted out of the rat race and didn't earn what he knew he was capable of earning.

What emerged during that first session was that Sam had issues of low self-confidence and self-esteem, which Elizabeth knew about but ignored and even exacerbated by her constant complaints and criticism. Elizabeth was a high achiever but felt she was not cherished and cared for as a woman, which led to her not feeling feminine in the bedroom. Her libido was low, but when she did feel sexy, the whole situation was tinged with resentment and anger so that she wouldn't allow either of them to enjoy the experience.

I asked them to close their eyes and each think of a real situation in which there'd been conflict, and spend a few minutes playing the scene over in their minds exactly as it had happened. Neither knew which situation the other had chosen. Elizabeth volunteered to share first while Sam observed with compassion. The only prerequisite was a commitment to honesty and to trying to find a mutually supportive solution.

Elizabeth described sitting at one end of the dining table in Sam's apartment with him at the other. She was tired, having just come from work, and resentful that Sam had been home for a couple of hours. Sam served the evening meal and sat down, and within minutes, an argument began. She was shouting at Sam and he was putting down his knife and fork, looking upset and hurt. She felt even more enraged by what she called his "victim look."

I asked her now to close her eyes and place herself somewhere in the visualization where she could view the situation as an observer. She chose to sit at a chair at the side of the table so that she could see both herself and Sam, and I asked her to watch the whole scene again. From this angle she could see much more of what was happening. "The woman" (herself) was already looking tired and angry even before she sat down to eat and the rest of the scene seemed inevitable. "The man" (Sam) was nervous, trying hard to make things special, but in doing so was almost obsequious in his desire to please and avert a problem. As the observer, she found that repugnant.

Now I asked her to clear the scene from her mind; then, with her eyes closed, to move for a moment into Sam's chair and to watch and feel the whole thing being played out again. Her eyes filled with tears as she reported what she saw and felt. He felt anxious and a bit jumpy, and was trying to cover this by cracking jokes and ignoring how tired the woman looked. The woman at the other end of the table was unappreciative of what he'd prepared, snarling in attack and quite frightening. From Sam's seat she could see that he was trying to avoid the attack and defuse the situation before it could begin by being as pleasing as he could.

We were careful then to make sure that Elizabeth was back in her own skin and well grounded before moving on to Sam, who'd been sitting enthralled at what was going on and having difficulty in refraining from comforting Elizabeth.

Sam closed his eyes and viewed the scene he'd chosen.

It was Sunday morning and he'd arrived at Elizabeth's apartment feeling warm and affectionate, hoping they could have a lovely day, perhaps make love. He'd brought some flowers and wanted to put them in a vase. She was cleaning the kitchen floor and he left footprints on it as he tried to get to the sink. Within no time there was an eruption. She was hurling accusations at him and he wished he hadn't come.

Sam then moved himself to a place in the visualization where he could see the whole scene again exactly as it happened. He chose to move to the other side of the kitchen and watch. "The man" (himself) looked like an eager child having arrived ready to play and looked crestfallen to find that his playmate was working. He tried to hide the look of disappointment and became tongue tied. "The woman" (Elizabeth) was trying to finish what she needed to do and was harassed by having to hurry to please the man and then by him clumsily making even more of a mess.

I then asked him to move into Elizabeth's shoes and view the scene again. With his eyes closed he was silent for a moment as he watched the scene from a different perspective. What he saw from her eyes was a carefree irresponsible child with little understanding of the pressure she was under from working hard all week, spending the evenings with him and catching up on her housework on the weekends when she was already tired. She was angry that he expected to just show up on her day off and play. He could see that the man was irritating both in his unwillingness to share the load and in his apparent disregard for her feelings.

After he had completely de-roled, we discussed what they'd found.

Each had gained insight into how they appeared to the other and what caused resentments that weren't openly discussed, but allowed to fester and spiral into inappropriately expressed anger, resulting in behavior that neither of them liked. If they were to make it as a couple, Sam needed to grow up and accept his share of the work in the relationship, and Elizabeth needed to lighten up and ask for help instead of resenting the fact that Sam hadn't read her mind. Their love wasn't in question, but their problematic communication and inability to deal with conflict assertively had almost cost them the relationship.

Though there was obviously more work to do, both individually and as a couple, eventually they set up home together again, in an apartment in which neither of them had lived before. Sam took a job commensurate with his creative talents as a designer. Because he loved to cook, he continued to do so while Elizabeth took on responsibilities that were more suited to her organizational skills. They agreed on a place where Sam could write and times when he would be undisturbed to follow his dream. They decided on a fair allotment of tasks and a regular time when they would go out and enjoy themselves and each other.

Most importantly they also set aside time together each week when they could have a look at what irritated them, what pleased them, what they needed to work on and what they needed to say to each other. The exercise of seeing it from the other's angle has remained a powerful tool for them. After the birth of their first child, Elizabeth moved to part-time employment and they managed to make ends meet. Sam is taking creative writing classes and continues to write his first novel.

Being Responsible and Honest— but with Kindness

Relationships demand responsibility. As we saw, when Sam started to take more of his share of the responsibility things got back in balance.

I'm 100 percent responsible for myself and for no one else except for children and sometimes the elderly and the sick. However, within *any* relationship there's responsibility *towards* the other—for the interactions with them, for the impact our behavior has on their life, to show up when we say we will, to keep promises, etc. Though it's other people's choice to do what they wish with what's said or done to them (their stuff, it's often termed), we need to be aware that what we do and say can be wounding, hurtful and cruel and we're responsible for how we choose to deliver our message. We need to be honest, but do it kindly.

For example someone could say to me that the color of the outfit I'm wearing doesn't suit me, the style is wrong and that I look dreadful. Or a gentler, kinder person could suggest that blue is my color and I look better with a longer jacket. The message gets through that the outfit I'm wearing doesn't flatter me, but the message is constructive and less wounding.

But what about the situation where you've said that things aren't good and need to change and the other person either doesn't hear or ignores you? Then perhaps you do have to spell it out in words of one syllable, but still kindly. Very occasionally however, a message needs to be delivered in its raw state for maximum effect. But choose those times with care!

Terri needed one of those confrontations.

She talked a lot about love, using the word freely about her friends and family. However, she was also eager to gossip, spread rumors and talk about people in a judgmental, negative fashion. She complained that her father was unkind to her mother and that her mother didn't deserve to be in that relationship. She said that her mother-in-law was unsupportive, rarely came to visit, had little to say when she did and rarely commented favorably on Terri's clothes. People at work didn't really know what they were doing and she could run the place better than her boss, if only she were given the chance. The employees at the bank were rude to her and the woman in the dry cleaner's had slighted her by not smiling when she handed her her change. She wanted to change her doctor because she felt misunderstood because he'd asked her to look at the real problem when she complained about backache for the sixth time in the last two years and all investigations had found nothing sinister.

Terri is an unhappy woman and will continue to be so until she stops focusing on all the perceived slights in her life and on the negative that she attracts to herself, and starts seeing the wonderful world she could create. What's more, she'll move from one relationship to another, starting off with unrealistic expectations of a fairytale ending, but feeling let down by everyone as eventually she relegates every potential partner to the garbage pile along with everything else in her life.

Most attempts to help her will be met with accusations that the other person doesn't understand, or with reasons why certain recommendations couldn't work in her case. Sadly, unless she's willing to take stock and look at her life realistically, take responsibility for herself and her actions, her thoughts and her attitude, she'll remain unhappy and isolated, genuinely feeling that she's unlucky and that life treats her badly.

In having the courage to tell her that, of course I'm now on the gossip list!

If you see some of Terri in yourself, stop for a moment and look round at all the good things you have. That won't make the others go away, but it will at least help you get things in perspective.

Having the Courage to Leave

Sometimes we expect too much from our mate. We're constantly developing and so are they, in a universe that's rapidly changing also. If you look realistically at who you are now compared with who you were say ten years ago, the chances are that you're quite different. Any partner you may have had then will have changed too. For some couples, their attachment and lifestyle ensures that they grow in parallel and therefore stay together, but for many, growth takes us off at a tangent and makes separation more likely. But this doesn't mean that, for a time at least, that partner was not perfect for us. It's good to acknowledge that there was a time, however short, of utter happiness and perfection from which we learned, gained and grew. If we can do this, the love that brought us together allows us to let go and part, and, though different, it can remain strong and wonderful still.

Though in times past people mated for life, and some still do, the pace of life has changed so much for both men and women, that unfortunately this becomes less likely. There's no shame nowadays in the fact that in a lifetime we may have more than one mate whom we love deeply and can go on caring for, though we may not stay physically together for the whole of our adult life. Perhaps the problem lies in promising to be together forever rather than in loving each other forever, for we can continue to love even though we may have to part. Ending relationships should not be approached lightly and effort should be made to hold fast if we can, especially where there are children involved. But if there comes a time when separation is the only solution, it can also be part of the love affair on which we've embarked.

Often partings are acrimonious and hateful. They don't have to be. It's not a fairytale that people can care for each other enough to part with dignity and love. However, if your partner needs some anger and even hate to help him leave, to help him catapult away from you so that separation is complete, then so be it. On a spiritual level it won't be so. From the highest level of you to the highest level of him there can still be light and healing. If you want a permanent separation, send light, at least for a while, till the scars left by torn heart bonds can heal without your being attracted to each other again with love. You'll find a meditation to help you with this in *The 7 Healing Chakras.*

Love isn't a prison. People do have a right to leave without suffering threat, indignity, violence or abuse. The bit of loving that people often don't mention, when asked what saying "I love you" means, is that part that grants freedom for the other to grow, whether or not that includes us. As the following poem by William Blake so eloquently illustrates, sometimes we fail to respect each other's freedom.

> *He caught me in his silken net,*
> *And shut me in his golden cage.*
> *He loves to sit and hear me sing,*
> *Then, laughing, sports and plays with me;*
> *Then stretches out my golden wing,*
> *And mocks my loss of liberty.*

"SONG" (1783)

Don't forget that one of the things you may be learning is how to take care of yourself by leaving. However, doing so before you've accepted that you're an active player in what's going on, is underselling yourself. You're part of the transaction, and played a part in the development of the scenario. Looking at our own part and accepting responsibility for it is empowering, making us someone to be counted rather than a victim who can change nothing and to whom life just happens. Whether you feel that you've been abused or have to accept that you did some of the abusing, you were playing the part simultaneously of giver and receiver and have been fulfilling your function, no matter how painful.

Divorce happens. And for some the grief of the loss is akin to that felt on the death of someone close. For some it feels worse, since the object of our affection is still alive but unavailable or hating us and living happily with someone else. Parting can leave us feeling hopeless and a failure, cynical about whether the relationship meant anything at all to the other. It did! And it did to you too. No matter what's happened in the end, the two of you had an experience essential to you both, which allowed you both to learn things that you wouldn't have learned in any other way. You gave to each other things that no one else could give. Your time together was unique. Though you parted, that too was part of the love story. There's no such thing as a failed relationship or a failed marriage. Every relationship is a success, even though some last for only a brief while.

But often we know for a long time that we need to leave and yet something still keeps us. It may be because we don't want to cause pain, create havoc in the lives of others, face the shame that we didn't make it or perhaps it's that we just haven't quite learned the whole lesson yet. But every day brings us closer to the inevitable and one day, it just happens. If you know you have to leave, hold onto that knowing while you gather the courage to go. It will happen when the time is exactly right and no one has the right to push you till then. Take care of yourself, honor your heart and do whatever you have to with kindness, fairness and a desire for the higher good of you both.

Recently I saw a beautiful painting. The caption read, "One day she got sick of hell and simply left."

Relations That Prevent Intimacy

Many clients I see are stuck in cages of sorts, often of their own making. The state of codependency makes a prison out of what could be love. Neither partner has the freedom to follow their own individual path. Such enmeshed relationships are seductive initially because of the promise of finding your "other half" and feeling complete. However, they're based on insecurity, fear and need. The outcome is almost invariably unhappy, with each feeling stifled but afraid to let go.

This pattern of relating is passed down within the family for generations till it's accepted as normal. The common accompaniments are separation, divorce, affairs, addiction of one kind or another and a great deal of unhappiness with little real intimacy. The following case history spans three generations in order to demonstrate the trans-generational nature of the problem.

Amy is unhappy and anxious. She's been depressed on and off for years.

Three years ago her daughter, Charlie, to whom she is very close, married Tony, after a brief courtship. Since then Amy had felt completely lost despite the fact that Charlie still telephoned every day and visited at least a couple of times a week. Her husband, Eddie, worked extremely hard and played a lot of golf. Amy suspected that he had the occasional affair, but really didn't want to know.

Amy's father was an alcoholic and Amy and her mother had been confidantes and best friends. In the second year of their marriage, Eddie gave up the struggle to compete with Amy's mother for time and attention and got more and more busy at work, spending more time socially with his clients and colleagues and building a life outside the home. Amy was almost relieved.

Their first child was a son, whom Eddie took under his wing. When he was old enough, Eddie took him off every weekend to play golf while Amy was at her mother's. Charlie was born four years later as Amy's mother's health started to deteriorate. Sadly, her mother died when Charlie was five, leaving a huge hole in Amy's life. Eddie was busy elsewhere and all of Amy's focus now fell on Charlie, who became the person in whom Amy would confide about her unhappiness in her marriage. The bond between them was a source of comfort for them both.

Over the last few months, Charlie's marriage had been less happy. Tony was spending less and less time at

home. From the beginning of the marriage he'd
complained about the amount of time that Charlie spent
either on the phone to her mom or visiting, and it had
become the kernel of most of the conflict between them.
She was now convinced that he was having an affair and
she didn't know what to do. The idea of divorce had arisen
in arguments and she was depressed and anxious. Amy was
really worried about her.

So what was going on here?

Well, we could go back years and find a similar pattern of
skewed relationships, the web of unhappiness spreading far and wide.
But let's see what we have just in these three generations.

In each generation there is tight, enmeshed bonding between
parent and child rather than husband and wife, preventing marital
intimacy and leaving the partners to try to get their needs met elsewhere, not necessarily in a sexual way, but with work, an affair, sport
or some addictive behavior. Charlie's husband is now finding the
same difficulties as her father did.

The men in this scenario are not hapless victims. Something
about their background allowed them to get tangled up in this—we
looked earlier at the similarities that bring us together. Nor is this
just a problem of relationships between women and their mothers.
Sons can be just as fiercely bonded to mothers and sometimes the
whole sibling group is involved. They attach strongly to one parent,
protecting her fiercely while rendering her more and more helpless,
preventing her from standing on her own feet and growing, and
sidelining the other parent, who eventually takes off with some other
interest and becomes the person seen by the rest of the family as "the
problem." New partners coming into the family may initially be attracted by what appears to be loving closeness, but eventually become
stifled and angry and either struggle for a while then leave, or get

into the same pattern of dysfunctional relating while the codependence spreads insidiously into the next generation. No one's happy. Relationships are held together by the fear of abandonment rather than love. There's acrimony, gossip and disharmony throughout and anyone who tries to bring the whole to a more honest and wholesome way of communicating will generally be scapegoated by the rest as the family closes ranks and rejects anything that might destabilize it. This goes for new prospective partners and therapists alike.

So what are they to do?

Well, unless Charlie is willing to divorce her mother, her marriage has little chance of survival. Amy needs help to properly grieve her mother and finally let her go, grow up, build a life of her own, either with her husband or without, and allow Charlie to have a chance of an intimate relationship, which hasn't been possible in their family for at least the three generations we looked at.

If some of this sounds familiar to you or if you feel scared or unwilling to look at your relationship and what simultaneously divides you yet holds you together, then perhaps you need to look at whether indeed your relationship is one of love or addiction. Acknowledging the existence of the addictive quality of our relationship forces us to acknowledge that something has to change and that's often the basic fear—that in changing there'll be more pain, loss, abandonment—that the separation anxiety will overwhelm us and that we will die. Fear locks us in and prevents us from stepping back, blowing the illusions, laying open to the light deceptions and games we've used for various nefarious purposes and defusing other methods of subterfuge. In fact our mode of relating not only to our significant other but often to the rest of the world needs to be challenged.

The good news is that only part of you is out of control. Part still copes and gets on with daily tasks. In speaking to that part, empowering it and acknowledging it we can start to feel strong, free and independent again. Though confronting the issue may be frightening, you'll be glad you did when you can breathe freely again and relate with love rather than fear.

What About Your Sex Life?

Sexual energy and spiritual energy are one and the same force. The passion that flows through you with love for the universe and the Divine is the same energy that can be given expression in human sexual love of your beloved. Sadly some people see spirituality and sexual passion as mutually exclusive. Your body was expertly designed to allow you to enjoy yourself in a multitude of ways, including erotic touch and sexual gratification. Trying to deny your natural sexual urges results in inner conflict that blocks your capacity to grow energetically in other ways. Sometimes, however, as spirituality becomes more developed there's a decline in the desire for sex with a partner since an ecstatic union within our own divinity is available.

It's a pity that sex has become associated with shame and guilt, with repression and rules that have frightened many of us about something that is the most natural thing in the world, and without which none of us would be here at all.

So, first let's look at sex.

It's been said that Don Juan was the greatest lover ever known. Rumor has it that for some years he had a different woman every night. But, perhaps the magic of the real lover is in being able to make love with the same person for years. To be aroused by their beauty still—even though the years may have jaded it. To be enchanted by the smile you fell in love with still—though wrinkles now replace the bloom of the peach. To allow the deep love you share to see beyond the physical and to tap the beauty that Antoine de Saint-Exupéry alludes to in *The Little Prince* when he says "what is really important is invisible to the eye."

There are great variations in what people refer to as sex. It's a far cry from sex of the mundane variety—that of the smutty joke, the nudge and the wink—to the powerful experience between two people who love each other, which can be akin to spiritual ecstasy. Though I'm sure there's a place for lusty sex, that's not the kind that I'm referring to here. Without the spiritual element, sex is a pleasant diversion, an erotic fantasy, but falls short of the holiness of transcendent sexual pleasure that's possible within the art of lovemaking.

Sexual love doesn't have to be part of the expression of love, though for most couples it is. There may be reasons why such sexual ecstasy isn't an option for some, yet their union can be tender and compassionate. There are more ways of making love than making love! Tenderness and a willingness to extend ourselves to pleasure the other can be as important as intercourse itself.

Sometimes due to illness, incapacity, emotional trauma or ill health sex is difficult if not impossible. Also some may choose celibacy—a lack of sexual gratification—within their relationship for a variety of reasons. Some young couples are once again making a contract to avoid sex before marriage, or at least until in a committed monogamous relationship, sometimes on religious grounds, but also on the back of the tidal wave of AIDS. Whatever the reasons, celibacy is a personal choice, though one that can cause difficulties if entered into unilaterally in the framework of an existing relationship. But where one partner does want celibacy as either a temporary or permanent state, it's something for the couple to discuss, respect and explore, though for many it would spell the end of the relationship.

Love can be genuine, adequate, nurturing and empowering without the act of intercourse. Sometimes as couples get older or have been together for a long time, the relationship becomes celibate quite naturally. Companionship, mutual support and desire for the other's well-being continue to sustain them.

Choosing celibacy on religious grounds, or as a means of self-sacrifice, demands great emotional maturity and interpersonal wholeness, since it doesn't necessarily mean that a desire for sex is absent and there's often still considerable inner struggle. Even within celibate relationships there can be rejoicing in the masculine and feminine that have come together in an inner marriage, both within each partner and within the partnership, and love and emotion can be expressed in different ways.

Improving Your Love Life

If you want to improve your love life, spend time with your partner exploring and exploding some of the myths you've both learned about sex, and which have formed a framework in which the two of you are trying to let go and relax into lovemaking. It's difficult to get to the state of abandon necessary to have an orgasm if your mind is stuck with old rules and beliefs, your body shut down with a paucity of energy flowing in any direction! Keeping such a discussion light and even humorous will enable you both to relax.

Sexual love can crown and transform you in a way that little else can, allowing the consummation of love and a completion of the union, with a feeling of becoming one in an emotional, physical and spiritual sense. It's a profoundly healing and nurturing experience. However, sexual love demands time and tenderness, compassion and celebration, understanding and reverence with a commitment, not necessarily forever, but certainly for the moment, to honor the other and desire their highest good. It contains an element of mystery, heightened by the depth of the connection between the couple.

If for some reason the two of you have had a break from lovemaking—perhaps one of you has been ill or depressed, or perhaps lovemaking has never really been established—take things slowly and go at the pace of the slower. Any attempt to rush things will usually result in further distancing. Perhaps the only intimacy possible for a while is hugging. A good idea, though not easy, is to commit to banning intercourse for some time. The two of you can get as close as you like, but the person who's afraid even to kiss in case it should lead to something else can get comfortable again. From this point perhaps you could move on to gently massaging each other, avoiding erogenous zones. (My patients laugh when I say, "No touching between neck and knees.") Eventually you'll probably slip into making love and enjoying each other. If, however, there's been serious trauma, assault or sexual abuse that is causing the problem, please get professional help for both of you.

Commitment—the Big "C"

Women are usually more inclined to want commitment than men, though sometimes the whole concept can be intimidating for either partner. The committed relationship can provide safety, trust, fulfillment, honesty and a nurturing nest where both partners can grow in love and sustain each other in every aspect of their lives. As I said earlier, perhaps the problem in making a commitment lies in promising to be together forever. Though that's a wonderful ideal, perhaps simply to love each other is a better one, for in that there can also be the commitment to let each other go if necessary; and, in the time you're together, to hold each other's higher good and transformation as an ideal for each of you and the relationship.

Commitment encompasses various areas of our lives together and it's wise for us to explore each other's expectations so that we know what we're committing to. Many relationships have fallen on the unspoken expectations and assumptions of the other! It's impossible to say how you're both going to feel five years from now, but

*Questions you might like to ask yourself
and each other*

*Do you both agree that monogamy is a good idea? Can you
both commit to honesty? Can you commit to being responsible
for yourselves and toward each other? Can you commit to allowing and even encouraging the other's growth even if that takes
them away from you? How do you feel about money? Are you
committed to sharing or having separate accounts? How do you
propose to split household chores? Are you both committed to
having children? Or not having children? How do you both feel
about spirituality? And religion? Part of the problem that arose
for Elizabeth and Sam (see page 223) was that because they
hadn't sorted out some of these basic issues each was hurt and
disappointed by the other even though they ultimately wanted
the same thing.*

certain expectations are probably not going to change and are fundamental. In days gone by, long courtships tested commitment—now
we try to take short cuts!

In order to make a responsible informed commitment, it would
be wise to spend some time looking at all of the questions above and
many more besides so that each of you knows what you're committing
to. Though it may seem like an unromantic exercise, just consider how
much you'll learn about each other and how many potential difficulties can be ironed out before they arise. If you really love each other,
neither the world nor your relationship will fall apart because you sit
down and are realistic about the future you're hoping to commit to.

Same-Sex Relationships

Though I feel that same-sex relationships need a mention, much of
what I've said goes for any combination of the sexes. People fall in

love, get into relationships, make commitments to each other and have deep feelings of joy, pleasure, hurt and pain, no matter what the combination of genders.

But if you're in a same-sex relationship, you'll know that you and your partner are subject to greater pressures than those in heterosexual relationships. Gay issues are much more in the open nowadays, yet there's still judgement and sometimes ridicule from families, friends, colleagues and society at large, which add extra strain. In the past at least, gay relationships often broke down under the stress of trying to survive in a vacuum, surrounded by secrecy. Happily the climate is changing and not only is it easier for gay people to find each other, but families are more likely to give their support and gay couples can have a circle of friends and live a more natural lifestyle.

You and your partner may have been deeply and lovingly committed to each other for many years with a depth of feeling similar to that of any heterosexual couple. You may feel that some celebration of your union is essential and decide to sanctify your relationship in a civil or church ceremony, or in a ceremony with close friends and family. There are some places where legal ceremonies are available, after which couples have similar legal rights to those offered to other married couples. However, there are still mountains to climb in terms of acceptance, individual and religious prejudice and rights that the rest of society take for granted.

You have similar access to spirituality and spiritual love and partnership whatever your gender preference. Heterosexual people don't have a monopoly on love. The God who some believe is sitting in judgment on gay people, despite the fact that all human beings were created in perfection, is human fantasy—a manmade illusion built on fear, which falls into the same category as the belief that those with different skin color are less perfect than the rest of us.

There's a wonderful book, *Is It a Choice?* by Eric Marcus, which answers a host of questions about same-sex love. *Permanent Partners* by Betty Burzon, Ph.D., is also a helpful classic.

And in the End . . .

We've looked at many aspects of loving relationships with partners, and I'm sure you're aware that we could go on forever. Be joyous in your relationship if you have one, and if you're still searching, open your heart and be still and ask the universe to do the rest. And if you have to leave, do so with honor and dignity, remembering that your most loving relationship is still with yourself.

Affirmation

*I open my heart and mind to the partner of my soul
with whom I have a loving commitment to the higher
good of us both. My heart flows with boundless love
and welcome.*

Meditation

Take yourself to your safe place and get comfortable. As you've done before, focus on your breathing and breathe in a feeling of tranquillity while letting anything negative simply drain out through your root chakra and the soles of your feet. Let your whole being be filled with light. Allow yourself to drift into a calm and serene state where there is peace flowing into and around you. See a white light falling around you, protecting you and holding you and nurturing you. Breathe in the light. Cleansing, healing, balancing.

Now take your focus down to your heart and allow the spinning green wheel of light to gently open. Spinning, spinning. See the pink light of love within your heart as it opens and let it spill into your whole body, nourishing you. Let it shine out now into your aura, bathing you in love, healing you. And now let it fall in a beam in front of you and there visualize your partner. If you have not yet met the person who is your partner, visualize a being who will be yours. Let the healing light surround you both.

Let the love from your heart reach out to your partner's heart and with tenderness and freedom, welcome them and wish them the highest possible good. Know that this love, radiating from your heart chakra, enriched by your crown, is the energy that renders you human while simultaneously demonstrating your divinity. This is the stuff of your soul and your connection with God. It enables you to forgive unconditionally, and to commune deeply with your beloved beyond what language can convey. Let them know that you wish for them happiness and health, the highest possible joy and peace. Tell them that your desire is for a love that enriches you both and helps each of you come to the fullness of your being. That between you there can be a devoted union—physical with physical; emotions with emotions; mind with mind; soul with soul, and that the love between you is a spiritual experience that will transform you both.

For as long as you wish, hold your beloved in the light and love, but with gentleness and lightness, not grasping or clutching. Remember that the more lightly we hold, the more people will choose to stay. Listen to any message you may receive and allow new insights to simply drop into your mind.

When you feel that it's almost time to return, allow your beloved to gently fade from your view and take the beam of love back into your heart. Feel yourself complete and whole, none of you left with your partner, so that the love between you can be independent and fresh.

Breathe in the beam of light in which you have been sitting and know that you remain protected. Gently close your chakras (see page 58) and when you're ready, start to be aware of your breathing and your physical presence. Move your fingers and toes. Return to a place behind your eyes and gently open them.

Stretch a little. Have a glass of water, check that you are completely grounded and record whatever you wish in your journal.

Nine

Beyond the Human—Loving Partnership with Our World

❧

Help me today to realize that you will be speaking to me through the events of the day. Through things, through people, through all creation. Give me ears, eyes and heart to perceive you, however veiled your presence may be. Give me insight to see through the exterior of things to the interior truth. Give me the spirit of discernment.

—Sir Jacob Astley, Battle Prayers

*I*n the previous chapters we've looked at relationships with people in our lives, and now we move to other loves: for the planet, our country, our way of life, animals and plants and for all with which we share the vast universe. In this chapter I want us to look also at our belonging in this time and space, and what we can do to preserve peace.

Intimate Relationship with All Things

There is no separation between us. However, our consciousness of that develops through stages.

In a spiritual sense, there's a time when we have individual consciousness, seeing ourselves as entirely separate from others. We've addressed this in earlier chapters. This is the level of development of our root chakra when we see ourselves as needing to survive, alone if necessary.

Eventually we come to accept that we're part of a group—we addressed this in looking at our relationships with family, friends and partners, though the group may be as broad as the human race. This level is known as group consciousness.

And now we move to a higher level of consciousness, what we might call Christ, Buddha or unity consciousness, where we feel our connection with the source of life, with all other life forms and all of the universe. In arriving at this level, we realize our intimate relationship with all things—that there's nothing on the planet with which we're *not* in an intimate relationship—whether human, animal, plant or mineral—and of course the earth itself and the atmosphere around it. Bringing this to conscious awareness can fill us with joy and awe, and also a great sense of responsibility as we see that whatever we do affects every single thing in the universe. And just as I can affect everything with a whisper, if I allow it, everything can affect me.

At this level of consciousness we see that neither time nor space separates us. The universe just *is*, in this eternal moment of now. Let's look at that concept a little more deeply.

As we saw in Chapter 2, there's no real space around us. We extend out into the universe, our subtle bodies moving ahead of the physical, affecting all that's around us. Our energetic body meets and mingles with others, sensing, giving us signals and preparing our way by sharing information about us.

Have you ever just paused in the moment of *now* and realized that no matter how still you are, you're constantly moving onward? Your body is carrying out its millions of chemical reactions, your cells are being born and growing, while others are reaching the end of their

A meditation of hope

A meditation of hope I often teach involves seeing ourselves at the tip of a rocket moving out into space, silently gliding through time, constantly, relentlessly moving forward into the future, leaving behind us all there ever was. No matter what we have done, or what has been done to us, no matter what we've been carrying and refusing to put down, the rocket keeps moving ever onward and yet its tip is always in the moment of now. We can choose to carry all our past along with us or we can jettison it since it no longer exists except in our minds. That can be so liberating. We need not carry baggage. The choice is ours. All of the things you've brought to mind in reading thus far—events of your childhood, your adolescence, family relationships from before you were born—simply let them all fall into space now, and move ahead free.

life and being recycled. There's constant motion. All around us there's similar activity that can never be stilled. And yet, when we stop and focus once more, we're still in the moment of *now*. The paradox is that though we cannot stop any living thing from moving onward, we're constantly in an endless moment. Every single thing that was when you started reading this sentence has changed. "Death" doesn't cause a ripple, a pause or a lost beat in the heart of the moment: everything continues to march on. We can never catch the next second, nor reclaim the last one. All that is past, no longer is. There is only this moment—*now*.

While I was writing this, I was flying from London back to my home in Texas and took a break to stretch and look out of the window. There below me on this wonderful late-October day, was broken cloud scattered across a landscape partially covered by snow with lakes iced over and rivers glistening like silver ribbons in the sunshine. Here and there clumps of fir trees stuck out of the snow, stiff and black in stark contrast to the softness of the snow and cloud. My heart opened even further with love and joy. Here am I in this moment filling my eyes, my heart and my mind with the beauty of the universe and here are you in this moment wherever you are on the planet and your heart and imagination can share that vision and that love. If that isn't wonderful, I don't know what is!

Just as this moment is neverending, so is this space in which I'm physically sitting writing this to you. And just as you're in this moment, you're in this space also. Here is my physical and auric body surrounded by a sea of molecules and somewhere, either close to me or afar, there's you. Your aura is mingling with the universal field too, and the vibrations between us join us no matter how much physical distance there is between us. There is no emptiness only a continuation of all there is. So whatever I do in this endless space in this endless now where you and I are not separate at all, I do to you and also to myself.

Whoever is in that space, whether I profess to love or hate them, is affected by whatever I do. Whether I'm happy and put out sweet love, or angry and put out bitter resentment, it touches everything. A soft whisper or a scream, a tender caress or the violent sweep of my arm through the air to hit, moves the "space" and, with a domino effect, affects all. Then, rather like a universal boomerang, it reverberates through the universe and comes back to affect me too.

Thus we are not individuals, nor merely a group, but are intimately and irrevocably linked, connected not only to each other but to all things.

Loving and Protecting the Planet

None of the earth can truly belong to any individual, country, government or power. Nevertheless, we do have the illusion of ownership. Each of us has the responsibility of taking care not only of the piece

The web of life

Chief Seattle, a peaceful, respected and inspiring chief of the Duwamish and Suquamish indians, born at the end of the eighteenth century in the Pacific Northwest, addressed our responsibility to the planet in his famous speech in the mid-1850s in Washington D.C. to the Commission of Indian Affairs for the Territory. This speech has been the basis of ecological movements around the world ever since.

He talked of the holiness of the land, the connection of the people with it and our responsibility to respect the earth, the water and the air, to acknowledge that they're essential to our well-being, supporting our physical life. "This we know," he said. "All things are connected like the blood that unites us. We did not weave the web of life, we are merely a strand in it. Whatever we do to the web, we do to ourselves."

of the planet that "belongs" to us, but also of all of the planet, by surrounding ourselves with peace and emitting peace.

The air that we breathe from our first gasp till our last breath is a living, swirling mass of gases, particles, molecules—of energy. Though the composition may have changed, it's the same air that has been breathed for centuries. We're also constructing our bodies of molecules that have been around for millions of years. The carbon atoms that are part of my body now are those that were part of the planet at its conception. They had been part of the body of millions of plants, animals and humans before they came to rest temporarily in me. And when they leave me, they will circulate once more. Whether we are animal, plant or mineral, only the way atoms are temporarily amalgamated distinguishes us. We're all made of the same stuff, literally, because physically, that's all that there is. The ever-changing sea of energy in which we live and of which we are made is in fact finite and eternal.

You may feel removed from the earth, in a city or in a high-rise apartment, but the earth is still yours. You can still claim part of it, even if only in having plants in your room.

Our Piece of the Planet

Though there are still wild open places which belong to us all and that none of us can own, many of us have pieces of land, however small, for which we have a responsibility.

When my sister and I were little girls, we each had a small area of the garden to call our own, which we would tend with small hand tools. We would plant seeds and be responsible for their growth. We learned to love the plants as they grew and with great pride we would then harvest what was ours. Tending our little part of the planet and helping it produce for us was a major lesson not only in self-sufficiency, but also in taking care of the earth and valuing the bounty it can produce.

Now as I walk in my pecan orchards and pick vegetables in my garden I have the same sweet delight in what the earth has produced. Raking and hoeing become combing the hair of the earth; watering, quenching her thirst; fertilizing, nourishing so that there will be an abundance come the harvest. Having part of the planet to care for is a privilege.

And what of our community land? If we love the planet, then parks, forests and hedgerows, lakesides, seashore and urban roadsides are sacrosanct too. Throwing litter, destroying trees and plants or vandalizing and polluting the earth with exhaust fumes, chlorofluorocarbons (CFCs), pesticides and other chemicals, becomes sacrilege.

So what can you do to help nurture the earth and reconnect with it? How can you take responsibility for part of the planet? Can you have a small vegetable plot? Can you take part in a conservation program? Or, if all else fails, perhaps you could grow some plants as the representation of the earth and its bounty.

Crystals

I love my crystals, use them in my work and my home, wear them, and feel a great connection with them. Over the years I've encouraged others to enjoy the benefits of these powerful gems. However, recently I've become quite concerned about the effect this must be having on the planet. There are millions of us now using crystals in one way or another, and shops and shows where thousands of crystals are on sale. Huge geodes have been dug out of the earth and it pains me in my heart to think of the gaping wounds that must be left in the planet. Added to this, of course, are the huge mining operations for other gems and precious metals, and even coal.

From time to time I return crystals to the earth in a special place and usually in a ceremony to mark some particular event. But perhaps I need to do more than that. In future, I will only buy crystals to use to return to the planet.

Perhaps you'd like to do the same and as the demand slows, the mining will cease and the planet need not be raped any more.

Patriotism and Our Roots

My mother used to recite a poem to me when I was young about a man turning his footsteps homeward and his heart burning for his native land. Unfortunately, I haven't been able to find the poem or its author, but I always loved it. Yet it only began to make sense as I traveled more, and though I see myself as a citizen of the world and have lived very happily on the African and American continents, more and more when I return to England, and particularly to County Durham, I have a lump in my throat as I revisit my roots and remember where I came from and why I chose this as my native land in this lifetime and all it has given me.

That is true of wherever you were born too. The planet in its wonderful variety of moods and landscapes has given you the start you needed. And though for some their time in that place may have been short because of war, chaos or other upheaval, the place from which we come is nevertheless one of the invariables we chose in reincarnating this time (see page 293). Somewhere in our hearts there will always be a connection, and in our souls loyalty and a feeling of patriotism, no matter how deeply that may be buried. At some time, usually when we're ready to do our root chakra work, no matter how informally, we revisit our roots. Some are unable ever to do so, physically exiled from their native land by politics, distance or finance, but you can visit it simply by looking into the depths of your heart and allowing your soul to reconnect.

As I said in Chapter 4, no one else shares your circumstances of birth, nor can they ever be changed. They're part of who you are, and are precious and to be valued highly. Though you may, like me, travel the planet, live elsewhere and take your inner home and your inner peace with you, the place where you began will never change. Value it and love it, no matter what the circumstances. The health of your root chakra depends on it, and thereby the stability of your whole life. Your love for your native land becomes part of your inner as well as outer world—part of your soul.

Patriotism and Loyalty

Though patriotism and loyalty to the place of our birth and the people who share similar roots are to be commended, for some they can become a barrier to integration into a new life and be the root of more serious problems of separation and discrimination.

Many expatriates, even after living in another country for many years, still hold allegiance to their roots, never fully embracing a new world. They stick together and keep to their original customs, language and culture. Many feel they had little choice in where they now live, and bringing with them their culture is proper and essential to their well-being. For the settlement and rehabilitation of refugees and other displaced persons, this is even more critical. However, it's sad to see that within some areas there's little or no integration, as though mingling would dilute and perhaps destroy a culture, with the loss of identity and moral values. Which, of course, it might.

Loyalty was originally to our kith and kin and perhaps to those in close proximity to us geographically, beyond which there was suspicion and mistrust. This allowed families or communities to hold together against attack and survive. In some parts of the world this is still so. However if loyalty is blind and narrow, it can become sinister and potentially dangerous.

Creating an "in" group, in whatever context, simultaneously creates an "out" group—those who are considered to be different, not part of us, and therefore separate and strange. This phenomenon can be seen in small ways within schools, business and family, and in greater ways within the world. Ties of loyalty between the members of the in-group can often lead to mistrust, suspicion and sometimes dislike of those in the out-group, though such feelings have no real basis since neither group really knows the other at all. Scapegoating begins and an escalation of negative feelings occurs until we have the nucleus of racism, victimization, gang warfare and full-scale war.

Individual expressions of this holding together against the outside world can be quite subtle, but then, at times of stress, develop quite rapidly into potentially explosive situations. This can be seen on a small scale or globally. The following demonstrates a quite subtle but nevertheless sinister development of such a situation.

Fairly recently a friend of mine was sad to witness painful events in a family to whom he was very close. What happened in the face of their pain however was both interesting and disturbing. It became obvious that, according to their family dynamics, someone had to be blamed for the events that had befallen them. Of course no one was to blame, but in order for everyone to settle and put the problem to rest, various people came under scrutiny to see what part they'd played in the development of the situation. My friend, as a loving outsider, offered care and sustenance to all the family members while grief and anger raged.

A few months later there was another, considerably smaller, family crisis. The previous feelings were resurrected, and once again the roving eye of blame began to search for a target. The first crisis had hurt them so much that the only thing they could do was to hold together even more strongly against the outside world, and the only one who was not part of that original nucleus was my friend. Despite the fact that he appeared to have been welcomed as one of their own, in fact he was the outsider. Suddenly, out of nowhere, he became the scapegoat for family disharmony that had existed for many years, allowing the actual blood relatives to hold each other in the "in" group and have an "out" group—my friend—upon whom to dump the negative feelings.

Imagine this on a larger scale—within a community where minorities are the "out" group; in countries where there are divisions on the grounds of color or creed. Here we have the nucleus of disruption of peace and potential disaster. For "loyalty" to our group, taken to its limit, causes division and brings our integrity into question. At the level of unity consciousness such divisions cannot occur, since we're all joined as one.

Is there some time in your life where you've created an in-group, with those outside the group being a target for suspicion or gossip? What about at work? In school? Are you part of a religious or racial group that protects itself against the rest of the world and therefore sets up a situation where those who are not of your group are left out? Does that benefit you? Or them? Is it really in line with your integrity? Look at the "holy wars" there have been and still are.

If you subscribe to divisiveness in any form, then you're only a few steps away from discrimination against the out-group.

The Slippery Road to Collusion

In a conflict between integrity and loyalty which is going to win? Do I loyally protect my child against authority when to do so calls me to be dishonest? Do you do your duty as a citizen when that means informing the police that your son is selling drugs to children? Do you make excuses yet again for why your husband is not at work when really it's because he's drunk? Do you tell the children to lie about how you got a black eye while punishing them for lying about other things? Whom do we become when passion and greed distract and preoccupy us? These are dilemmas that bring our loyalty into conflict with our integrity and show how, when misplaced, loyalty can become an ominous tool.

Taken further, we can see how misplaced loyalty creates divisions and leads to situations where normal morality, common sense and decency get lost in bigotry and fanaticism. Ethnic cleansing, apartheid, slavery and child labor probably outrage most of us, while we may turn a blind eye to lesser variations of the same lack of love when someone's teased and scapegoated in school or office till their life is made a misery. Or when snide comments about those of a different race or color go unchallenged by us because we haven't the courage to stand against those with whom we're generally allied. When we see children being misused in the supermarket or animals being neglected and do nothing. When we listen to the gossip and add our own bit and allow the systematic assassination of someone's character. Our "loyalty" to our group gets in the way of what we know is right, or we get carried along with the crowd without stopping to think what our true stand on the matter is. We're afraid to be seen as different, to be called "goodie goodie" when we refuse to gossip with others. In fact, we are afraid that we too may be relegated to the out-group. Those who followed Hitler had a similar problem.

Such moral issues call us to make decisions with our hearts on the basis of love, empathy, compassion and integrity. But what we may see as authoritative sources often give ambiguous and ambivalent messages on such issues. We only have to look at the politicians' stance on accepting enormous revenue from the tobacco industry while knowing that it's collected on the back of millions of deaths. Throughout the world while most religions have preached about the brotherhood of man, both the Koran and the Bible appear in places to condone slavery. And apartheid is seen by some to have the blessing of the Bible. Despite this, we've moved almost en masse towards an awareness of universal equality. To some this is still simply an intellectual exercise. With the development of a higher level of consciousness, such issues are very clear.

This development of the heart chakra is moving us towards a more enlightened way of being. We're bonded together as members of a universal family, a huge body of humanity. We are part of a collective consciousness, held together by a common decency that prompts most of us to act as we intuitively know we should. It's to this universal family that we owe loyalty. Here we can find a system of beliefs and social norms that will encourage us to live peaceably together. Here bonds of love and loyalty will ensure that our children are happy and safe and that the sick, the elderly and infirm are cared for.

Taking Care of Now—Protecting Our Peace

Light and sound waves go on for ever. Whispers and loving words of centuries ago still reverberate in the universe now. So do angry words and screams. Since we're constantly recycling all there is, it continues to affect us subconsciously and becomes part of the fabric of our lives. It's not only noxious fumes, but noxious attitudes, feelings and words that disturb our peace and pollute our world.

It's expedient then to be responsible and careful about what we release into the universe. The careless remark, cruel jibe, anger and violence will reverberate forever. They are the fodder and fuel of our future, that of our children and of all those as yet unborn. So it would be responsible to state our feelings kindly when we can.

If we were to imagine the universal "space" as a garden, we could plant it with music, peaceful chants, harmonious sound, sweet words whispered into the breeze, prayers breathed out to God and laughter. The sound of wind chimes and the song of birds to soothe our world. And silence!

Peace is our natural state, and we have a responsibility to protect and preserve it. Therefore being aware of what takes us out of our peace, and making wise decisions about where and with whom we wish to be so that we can remain peaceful, ensures that our contribution to the planet is gentle and loving.

Doing the work that I do, I need to be in peace. That's not me being precious, it's simply an active choice. I choose to have my heart lovingly open to embrace the universe and all its wonders in an atmosphere of calm. I want to breathe easily without having to protect myself. I want to have the space round the tip of my rocket as clear and loving and peaceful as I can possibly make it so that I can drift on into eternity, enjoying the wonder of every sight and sound with my heart and mind free. That means I have to make responsible choices, some of which might not be very popular.

Generally I choose not to have the media throwing violence and garbage into my sitting room or onto my breakfast table. Neither I, nor my home, nor the people and animals that share my home needs that. I don't want people to pollute my world either! So relationships need to be loving, mutually respectful and nurturing. That begins with me respecting myself enough to think about and state what's right and acceptable for me. And if, in the main, relationships cannot be peaceful, based on trust, love and honesty, I need to work on them as hard as I can, and then, if necessary, make the decision to let them go in love and dignity. Those with whom we cannot have mutual respect and peace, love and laughter, disrupt our harmonious soul connection with God, while we disrupt theirs.

Even then, since there is no space between us, they can still be affected by us and we by them, though often to a lesser degree. Whatever was disturbing us both is likely to do so less if we're not in each other's physical presence, caught up in convoluted communication that's been impossible to change. Separation, though painful, often allows us to reclaim our peace and our soul, which becomes fragmented in the chaos of constant argument and anger. This conscious decision is neither running away nor opting out, but valuing ourselves and them, and placing love, peace and our connection with our spirit above all.

It's also our responsibility to minimize distractions to peace in the universe. We can do this by putting out love to neutralize anger, fear, resentment and hatred; flowing love into politicians so that they accept divine guidance and make decisions that will move us all towards peace; persuading others that guns and weapons are not an option and that we can disarm and yet empower ourselves and others with love. We need to get the message out into the world that taking up violence in any form is not a solution. Perhaps you'd like to use the meditation at the end of this chapter to add your own power to this end.

And If There Has To Be Negativity . . .

Although I love to live in peace I've also chosen to work with many wonderful souls for whom peace is elusive, whose lives are shattered

Anger—things to remember, things to try

- It's human to be angry sometimes and hard to contain the energy that needs to erupt.
- In the heat of rage it's easy to hurl it at the perceived cause of our pain. Try not to.
- The energy you expel goes on forever, touching not only those around us at the time, but everything else also, making buildings as well as people sick. Anger lodges in our energy fields and those of others.
- When we're angry we perceive anger everywhere as it spreads around us like a pervasive gas; then we pick it up again as though it doesn't belong to us.
- Children are particularly susceptible to atmosphere and cannot avoid anger—if you're angry and upset, your children will be fractious and everything appears to go wrong.
- Try to externalize anger with activity—exercise, gardening, cycling or having a really stomping walk on the earth.
- Go somewhere alone and have a tantrum, beat your bed, scream into your pillow.
- Put on some music and move to it, eventually building up to a powerful dance that can externalize your fury.
- Feel the power in your anger and use it constructively to plan positive change—though don't act on it until you're calm again.
- Write letters you're not going to send to those you perceive as having made you angry.
- Own the anger—it's a powerful energy that is yours and you can learn to redirect it and use it to effect change in your life.
- Read some books on dealing with your anger, for example, Ten Basic Steps to Managing Your Anger, W. Doyle Gentry; Anger: Deal with It, Stop It from Killing You, Bill Defoore; Overcoming Hurts and Anger, Dwight L. Carlson, M.D.
- If you have persistent anger to the point of fury or rage, think of seeking professional help.

by pain. The only way I can cope with the pain and negativity that often surrounds them is to protect my heart chakra and constantly flow love outward. In this way, I can usually hold my peace and love endlessly, despite what might be released into the space in which I work. If you're doing such work, or find that at work or home, for now, you cannot escape negativity, do protect yourself well. Working with angels, guides and helpers is essential to me. We'll talk of that again in the next chapter.

What we can do while working and being adequately prepared is more difficult at home, where your emotions are involved in a different way. If you feel stressed out or unwell, look at where you need to protect yourself better and also at how you're going to reduce the stress in your life. You deserve to have peace, though if you've had chaos for so long, you might find it difficult to know what to do with it!

But don't feel too bad! Those who are working with negative energy in order to transform by dealing with the darker aspects of themselves (and that includes us all, to some extent) need there to be negativity in the universe at this point in time. It's part of the natural balance, though hopefully there'll be a time when we're beyond it. The task of the last generation was to deal with conflict by having great wars. In this generation our task is to help move to a higher consciousness.

Some generous souls have opted to work with negative energy to show us the way *not* to go—so that we can learn without having personal experience. We have learned about the horrors of war and why we should avoid it because of those loving souls who went ahead of us and experienced it for us. We know that we should work to free children from slave labor because both the children and those who enslave them have lived out that horror for us to see. We know that murder and torture are abhorrent because of those who have sacri-

Professional loving

Doctors, nurses, professional careers of children, the ill and the elderly, therapists, social workers, those in the probation service and countless others are engaged in professional loving day by day. We extend ourselves for the benefit of our clients while retaining a professional boundary that allows us to love with detachment. But we truly love, nevertheless.

I extend myself to give my patients what they need (which might be different from what they say they want), support where I can, delight in their achievements and grieve with them in their losses. I set limits with love, being firm where necessary, and challenge behavior that others who may have loved them differently have allowed to continue to their ultimate detriment. When the time comes, I lovingly let them go, wish them well and watch from a distance as they make their way in life. I still love them when they reject what I say, when sometimes they use me as a scapegoat, blame me for having broken a marriage (could I be that powerful?) or for not having been there enough. When they would love to stay in the warmth of a loving relationship with me I love them enough to push them out of the nest and into life. I'm aware that for some people shifting dependence from one thing to another as a stepping stone is part of the healing process. Sometimes I'm that stepping stone. I have no expectation of mutuality, no demand for them to love me, though often I know they do—and the richness I gain is immense. I give them freedom to make their own decisions and to realize their potential and become the best that they can be. This relationship with my patients therefore meets all the criteria of love. It's not just about "doing my job"; it goes far beyond that.

It would be wonderful to teach professional loving as part of the curriculum to other training professionals. Some in the prison service, for example, do actually love those in their care, but many more could learn to communicate to the best rather than

the worst aspects of people. There are politicians who are professionally loving and altruistic, but more who could learn to see
peace rather than profit as a prime goal, focusing more on harmony in the world than on developing weapons, more on feeding the hungry than preserving revenue and quotas.

Professional functional loving requires great discipline of the
heart chakra, and those involved in jobs where we use our
hearts in caring for others need support and supervision for the
benefit and protection of all. Some, afraid of the strength of their
own feelings, divorce themselves from their emotions in their
professional lives, but much is then lost to the client in terms of
warmth and the loving energy of another human heart. Many
would find it nearly impossible to do what they must professionally if they allowed themselves to have feelings for their clients.
There's a beautiful poem that looks at the difference between
doctors who wear their white coats and keep their hearts hidden and others who work with their hearts but can then get
hurt. But as Mother Teresa said, "I have found the paradox that
if I love till it hurts, there is no more hurt, but only more love."

As author Thomas Merton said, "Love seeks one thing only: the
good of the one loved. It leaves all other secondary effects to
take care of themselves. Love, therefore, is its own reward." A
teacher who loves her students, a nurse who loves her patients,
a healer who loves those for whom she is channeling healing,
expects nothing in return. But since all transactions are two-way
streets, we learn wherever we teach and receive, wherever we
give. What a blessing!

If you're in a profession that leads you to struggle with such
matters, why not talk it over with someone or set up a support
group within your facility. Sadly, this is an area that many refuse
to confront or discuss for fear of being seen with disapproval as
"too involved."

ficed themselves that we may be witnesses to their suffering and turn away from violence.

It's because we're all intimately joined—all part of the cosmic web—that we can teach and learn in such a way.

Loving Connection with Animals

Most of us who have experienced living with a dog or cat will be aware of the strong tie that develops with the animal—feelings that have the hallmark of true love.

In his remarkable and unique book, *Kinship with All Life*, J. Allen Boone describes simple yet challenging real life experiences showing how animals communicate with each other and those who understand them. He describes the often silent exchange of information that takes place between animal and human when we're willing to be flexible and receptive, to see the animal as an equal part of the universe and an expression of the universal mind just as we are.

He talks of a language of the heart and mind that requires no sound and is nothing to do with brain function but is "more authoritative . . . with all the immensity, all the power, all the intelligence and all the love of the mind of the universe moving in it and through it." From a sense of wonder at the communication he was able to have with a dog, he theorizes about the possibility of similar interplay with other life forms, concluding that the same force works through all living things in a "ceaseless rhythm of harmonious kinship."

Such communication with animals demands mutual respect, admiration, appreciation and courtesy as well as a desire to share the best aspects of ourselves and the best level of information we can with the other. Only when spoiled by human attention do animals behave with less than pure heart and motive. We can choose to communicate with them seeing ourselves as the master and the superior race, or we can assume a different perspective. The depth of love we can reach with animals is enhanced by educating our animal rather

---

Use your dog as a model . . .

If all else fails, just look at what you can learn from the behavior of a beloved dog! Dogs run to greet loved ones who return home, are loyal, never pretend to be what they are not, love to touch and be touched. They tune in when you have a bad day and sit silently, nuzzling you now and then for reassurance. They never hold grudges or pout, and they delight in seeing their friends. They show appreciation for a good meal and enjoy nothing more than having a lovely, long walk in the country with you. In general, they just enjoy being alive and will show you that by wagging not only their tail but their entire body. Now tell me that animals have nothing to teach us!!

---

than training it simply to behave exactly as we demand. A totally different, exciting relationship is then possible, in which a new kind of love exists.

Native Americans embrace a friendly identification with all life and a personal respect for the planet and all that lives and breathes upon it. They recognize that while the physical part of us walks the earth, there is a mental and spiritual part of us that moves in boundless space. In respecting that all things share this boundless space and time, the Native Americans develop a sense of kinship with everything from animals to the wind and the earth, talking of all of them as brothers and ancestors. They appear to refer to the universe metaphorically, but they believe profoundly in the presence of ancestors within the souls of living things and even the land, and talk of them with deep love and respect.

Loving Connection with the Plant Kingdom

Some of my dearest memories of my childhood are of wandering in the fields naming the flowers and collecting a bunch to take home.

As more children grow up in urban areas, even though councils do a great job with parks and recreation areas and planting on municipal ground, many have lost or never had the opportunity for a connection with the energy of wild and ancient trees and flowers strewn in grassy fields. Some never even see fresh fruit and vegetables. But we're intimately connected with the plant kingdom and need to honor and respect it in a way similar to that in which we respect animals and human life. Plants keep us alive. Oxygen comes from the natural metabolism of plants and they keep manageable the levels of other essential gases. Plants perfume the air while cleaning it of pollutants. Trees cleanse city air of exhaust fumes in a way that nothing else can.

The food chain starts always with the plants of the earth. They give us neatly packed energy and a whole array of vitamins and minerals essential to our well-being. They also provide us with herbs for medicinal and culinary purposes. Trees give off remarkable energy. I used to suffer much ridicule from my colleagues for introducing my depressed patients to an oak tree where they could sit or stand and gain comfort. Even if you can't physically feel the energy, give it a try. If you're feeling vulnerable, stand with your back to an oak tree, or better still hug it and allow yourself to simply breathe with it and see what happens. You might be amazed.

Healers for thousands of years have honored the sacred balance of the natural world. Herbal medicine is perhaps the oldest form of healing. Many of the pioneers of such healing were labeled witches and charlatans and suffered horrendously for their beliefs. There have always been the wise women of countryside communities who orally hand down their knowledge of how to collect herbs and use them to treat the sick. The modern pharmaceutical industry has developed from these beginnings. Thankfully there's currently a move away from synthetic drugs again and a demand for more natural remedies to treat illness and to bolster our well-being. Many of these can be found in *Total Wellbeing* by Dr. Hilary Jones and Dr. Brenda Davies.

Using the natural bounty of the earth, carefully and wisely, invites a sense of the divine into our daily lives. Leaving places that are wild and natural—a habitat for wildlife and a sanctuary for butterflies—is a gift to the earth, but also to yourself. Spend a little time appropriately dressed in the country, suspend your cynicism and judgement and just see what happens to your level of energy and your mood. I assure you that your heart chakra will open and your root chakra will become more balanced and though you may find emotions emerging that you had forgotten or repressed, the outcome will be greatly to your benefit.

Actively Doing Good and Minimizing Harm—a Different Way

So what can we do to ensure that we actively do good and not harm?

First of all we can be responsible with our own energy. We can endeavor to put out into the world only what is loving and kind. When we feel anger we can deal with it appropriately. And we can send loving, peaceful energy to those who are angry and in pain, feel resentful and violent or are suffering angst, to help them calm and transmute the energy they're feeling. In this way anger and hatred will eventually subside.

We can choose gentle energy. We can choose to affect our neighbors positively by thinking pleasant thoughts about them—sending loving mind messages that will touch and heal them. We can refuse to listen to or pass on gossip and hurtful comments. The perception that violence can only be dealt with by violence, that the old law of an eye for an eye is valid, remain obstacles to true peace. As long as we buy into that in any form, we're part of the crime and equal perpetrators.

In the summer of 1999 the beautiful, sleepy little town in Texas that is closest to my ranch was shattered one Sunday morning when the pastor and his wife were found bludgeoned to death in their bed.

Two weeks later, a quiet widowed grandmother was similarly murdered only a couple of miles away. For the next few weeks, as further murders came to light, the whole community became locked in fear and sadness.

The town was simultaneously amalgamated and split by what had happened. Joined by pain, shock, suffering and loss, they clung together in memorial services and in grief. But some bought guns to protect themselves, put up fences and lived in fear and others put into practice the truth that they had professed in church every Sunday of their lives, and often in between: that they would love their brother as themselves and that we are all one in the sight of God.

Many of my friends around the world joined with me in regular meditations for peace and to infuse the whole situation with love. The perpetrator of the crimes obviously didn't have enough love or he would not have behaved in such a manner. Sending him anger and hate would only inflame the situation. Isolation, fear and lack of love had driven him to such extreme acts and only the opposite of that could stop him. Sending him love and angels to protect him so that he wouldn't hurt anyone else or himself prompted ridicule from some, but in fact was the most logical way to deal with the situation. When, five weeks later, he surrendered himself, those of us who'd been focusing never-ending love on him, guiding him out of the confusion in which he had been living, rejoiced, but sadly, many would have stood by with lynching ropes had he not been protected by the law.

With love we can help change the anger and pain that cause the terrorist to pick up a gun or the murderer to raise a weapon. With a smile we can help another shift his mood from sadness to delight. With gentle and loving persistence and active self-management, we can help end the pollution of the atmosphere. We can move mountains, change the constitution of our own cells and to some extent those of others by spreading love around us and flowing it into those we meet. The energy of everything that is in my sphere can be directly changed by my love. By flowing a stream of never-ending love in all directions, we can change the world.

It's been said that this could be seen as an assault by those who don't believe in such things. However, we cannot stop the ceaseless flow of energy between us—that's just the way it is. Whether we like it or not we're affected by others, so we might as well, with good intention, put out into the world peace and love: then at last we can have a positive effect instead of a negative one.

A word of love and caution: none of us is peaceful all the time. Even with the best of intentions we get angry and say and do things it would have been better if we hadn't. Be gentle with yourself. If we were perfect there'd be no need for us still to be here. We're all making it by trial and error.

To a More Loving and Peaceful World

Each of us has chosen to come into the world in a position where we can do our best work, whether it be to affect the lives of millions or gently to show love to the close circle about us.

Our energy has impact on everyone, but especially on the lives of those with whom we actively interact. Some people are drawn to interact with huge numbers of people and enhance millions of lives. Entertainers, for instance, have chosen such a responsibility. Sometimes not only their talent but the example of their lives are gifts to their followers. For example Tina Turner, who is not only a talented performer but has demonstrated emergence into spiritual peace having survived enormous personal pain; Richard Gere, a great and inspiring actor who uses his spirit and his place in the world to extend the struggle for the freedom of Tibet; Shirley MacLaine, actress, dancer, comedian, who risked writing about her spiritual beliefs at a time when such self-disclosure might have invited ridicule. Look at Mother Teresa who in her simple and unflamboyant way changed the consciousness of the world. These are souls willing to sacrifice their privacy and use their human gifts to raise the level of consciousness of the world.

Most of us have chosen a different though equally important route for raising consciousness and bringing love and peace to the world. We've invested our loving energy in smaller spheres, but similarly change the consciousness of those around us. The parents who demonstrate love to their children affect not only their family. As the children enter the world, they in turn carry that message forward to whomever they meet and eventually to the next generation. Teachers in schools and colleges help young people uncover their knowledge and gifts and spread them farther afield. The person who takes away our refuse, and who does it with dedication to clearing and cleaning our environment, performs a necessary and worthwhile task that beautifies our planet. Everyone in any walk of life who performs their life's work in a spirit of joy and service brings life and energy to the rest of us and thereby promotes peace.

Souls who come from a position of love, who have raised their own consciousness and can see themselves and the world with clarity, compassion and wisdom, who have accepted their own inner power, have stretched themselves to become the best that they can be, in whatever sphere, are spreading vibrations of love which encompass the whole universe.

Affirmation

The following poem by James Elroy Flecker is a wonderful affirmation:

> *Since I can never see your face,*
> *And never shake you by the hand,*
> *I send you my soul through time and space*
> *To greet you. You will understand.*

Meditation

Take yourself to your safe place and make yourself comfortable. Concentrate for a moment on your breathing and allow peace and light to enter into you and fill your aura as you breathe out any anxiety and simply let negativity drain out through the soles of your feet and your root chakra. Visualize a white light shining down upon you protecting you, holding you in love and peace.

Now focus on your heart and allow it to open and, with a breath, fill every part of you—your physical body and your aura—with love. Let it heal and balance every bit of you, bringing you to a state of harmony and peace. Breathe into it and enjoy.

Now let your love spread around you and neutralize any anger you have felt recently. Let it heal your solar plexus where old feelings are stored. Allow the love of forgiveness to heal old pain and resentment and let go of anything you no longer need. All that is of the past has gone. It no longer exists. Let it go and in its place let there be love and light.

Feel your consciousness rise now. See yourself in a never-ending sea of love surrounding you and everything in the universe. Explore this vast universe of which you are an integral part. There is no separation between you and any other thing. Feel the love of other beings that surround you, their energy mingling with yours. Bid welcome to all that you acknowledge for the first time to be part of you. And in this moment commit yourself to love. To loving the universe and all its wonders. To the deepest oceans and the highest mountains. To lost valleys and islands. To shanty towns and urban areas. To the farthest corners of the universe, breathe your love. Commit yourself to preserving peace among all things. To protecting the rights of all. To protecting the health and beauty of all. To supporting the fulfillment of potential in all areas of the planet in line with the laws of nature and the universe.

Across time and space let there be only love.

Stay as long as you wish and enjoy.

When you're ready, come back into your body. Be aware of your breathing. Allow your heart chakra to gently close to a point where it feels comfortable and start to be aware of your physical presence. Move your fingers and your toes and feel your connection with the earth. Return to a place behind your eyes now and when you're ready, gently open them.

Stretch a little. Have a drink of water and when you're ready, record whatever you wish in your journal.

Ten

Divine Love

❦

*It were wiser to speak less of God, whom we cannot under-
stand, and more of each other, whom we can understand. Yet I
would have you know that we are the breath and the fragrance
of God. We are God in leaf, in flower and oftentimes in fruit.*

—KAHLIL GIBRAN

Like the universe, we're constantly in a state of flux. As parts of
us evolve, others are recycling; parts of us are stable while others struggle for balance; parts of us are increasing in sophistication
while others return to utter simplicity. In every second we're both
poised for action and resting. But, also mimicking the universe, the
whole is in magnificent equilibrium, a wonderful microcosm within
the macrocosm.

As I said in the introduction, what I call God, you may know
by another name. The ultimate Being is the same.

The Wilderness That Changes Our Lives

In every human life, and indeed the life of nations and of the planet
itself, there's a time when we feel as if we are lost and wandering in

the wilderness. It's a painful time, and often one that we fear will have no end. But it's an essential time of metamorphosis and, like the butterfly, we can emerge beautiful and brilliant. To get the most out of our own experiences, however, and to teach the maximum to others by them, we must perceive them correctly as great gifts that help us move towards a state of enlightenment.

In the late 1970s I returned to England after having lived in central Africa for some years with my husband and my two children. Though the sojourn in Africa was one of the most wonderful times of my life, in some ways, looking back, I can see that it also prompted my time in the wilderness. I learned a great deal and had extraordinary experiences, but in comparison to before and after that period, I neglected my spiritual life in favor of a more hedonistic adventure.

Our return to England was precipitated by a painful time. I look back on the severe depression that I suffered not long after our return as one of the greatest gifts of my life. It shaped me and intensified my compassion for the suffering of others in a way that no pleasant experience could have done and it allowed me to rise from it a better person and with new coping skills with which to face the world. But more than that, it allowed me to teach in a different way. First of all it gave me firsthand experience of the suffering of depression, and it allowed me to show others that there's a way out and that we needn't be damaged by the experience, nor bitter because of it. It enabled me to be an example to others of how to deal with emotional pain—to slide into it without resistance knowing that in the long run we're safe, held in love by God and the universe, and that whatever may happen to our physical being, our spirit continues to survive—and not only survive, but be strengthened by having been tempered by life.

That's not to say that while I was in the depths of my illness I didn't sometimes give in to despair. I did. I thought many times that death would be better than having to live through such pain. If I

hadn't had children whom I love dearly and for whom I felt a sense
of responsibility, and parents who would have suffered terribly from
my death, then I cannot say that I would not have succumbed to the
temptation to opt out of life. But having survived, I can see the great
benefit of such pain. I moved into the study of psychiatry from my
first love, surgery, and I know that that is where I was always meant
to be. In effect, being depressed changed my life for the better, and
I thank God for having had the experience.

The reawakening of my soul quickened, and far from feeling
abandoned, I felt a deepening connection with the universe and with
God. My depression made sense of the whole experience of life: that
we're tested and our physical being may appear damaged but that our
spirit continues to grow in strength, reaching ever closer to the God
from which we came and of whom we're forever a part. Suffering
intensifies our living, not our dying. In its clearest interpretation, it
is a call for us to move on in peace rather than in turmoil, and we do
have a choice.

Those who may have prompted you to move into a depressed
stance, those who appear to have assaulted you and done you harm,
are merely instruments to bring you the gift of a new lesson for which,
from the point of the purest love and forgiveness, you can be grateful. Your spiritual awakening is your resurrection—opening your
mind to what you already know and have always known: that your
task is to give and inspire love.

In Search of God

In each of us, often unrecognized and unnamed, is a profound longing, a yearning, to be united once more with the force we may call
God. This passion deep within our heart and soul calls us magically
and mysteriously, guiding our lives until we submit to its indescribable bittersweet longing. It's almost an indescribable grieving for some-

thing we can't reach—rather like homesickness or nostalgia. It calls us to become all that we can be despite how impractical, improbable or absurd our aims may appear to others. It keeps us going through disappointments and stumblings, our spirit fixed on a distant beacon that we simply know we must follow. *Pothos* (see page 43), the call of God, the siren drawing us not to the rocks but to blissful reunion with that divine part of us that we forgot in our quest to be human.

Sometimes subconsciously and sometimes with great conscious longing, we continue to search until we find it again. For some that may take a lifetime. Some may feel they never find it and spend their days in tortured wandering, missing out on the joys that are in every moment, lacking recognition that God is in every second, every transaction, every human face, every gesture, no matter how mundane or apparently profane. For in fact there's nothing but God, though in a million disguises, each giving a different gift, broadening our experience and bringing us back to wholeness.

Spiritual Connection and Inspiration

Though for much of our lives we may not be aware of it, we're always connected to God with our soul via our spirit. If we can remember this, nothing else matters. Therein lies immortality. Only the material manifestation of who we are at the moment can be harmed.

As we discussed in Chapter 4, my body allows me to manifest concretely so that I can exist here as a human being. It allows me human experience and I have a responsibility to cherish and take care of it so that it will serve me well and not divert my attention from the more important things I came here to do. The recognition of the mortality of my body and the immortality of my spirit allows me to be free from concern about what we call death and get on with living until I've completed what I came to do and will be released to be a free spirit again. No matter what may befall this human part of me, my spirit will go on and return to the body of God.

It also releases me to see whatever befalls me not as punishment but as an opportunity to grow in transaction with those who have agreed to be with me on this part of my journey and share the experience. Though on a human level it may appear that I'm a victim, I'm also teaching the other what it's like to be a perpetrator. We're equal students in an agreed contract, giving and receiving wisdom, experience and love, playing out ancient pacts made together by souls who know and love each other.

Recognizing ourselves as coming from, and being part of, God allows us to perceive our own greatness and that of every other soul around us. Now the world changes! From such a spiritual perspective there is equality, perfection, joy, peace and most of all great love, even though we're still striving to understand the lessons we came to learn and in doing so continue to generate inequality, imperfection, unhappiness, disaster and pain.

A great philosopher once said that when we are inspired by some great purpose or extraordinary project, dormant forces, faculties and talents come alive and we discover ourselves to be capable of much more than we ever thought possible. As the spirit flows through us we move from the human level where we can share intelligent information to a different plane where the spirit speaks and inspiration flows from us.

But inspiration requires that we keep open the channel of communication between ourselves and God—that is that we keep open our spirituality. To do that we need an open heart chakra and an open crown with the channel between free. We can do this partly by remaining open to the wonders of creation, and seeing the love explicit in everything around us. We must also be willing to see with loving eyes and without judgement, to give unconditionally, to see others as

our perfect equal no matter where they are on their particular journey towards enlightenment and to be willing to both learn and teach
in every transaction with others.

Reaching God

For centuries, devout people have devised rituals to help them open
up their connection and reach God. Burning incense and anointing
with oils are still common practices. However, though rituals can be
useful, and some are therapeutic, it's important to recognize that
they're only an aid and not a necessary part of the spiritual process.

Spiritual connection occurs anywhere, any time. We need neither priest nor guide. God is waiting for you everywhere and longing
for you to truly connect again whether you're walking on the beach,
sitting under a tree, lying in bed or sitting on the sofa. Nothing is
required except the willingness to connect. Any disconnection I feel
is my doing. Recently outside a church I saw the following banner:
"If you feel you can't reach God anymore, who moved?" All I need
to do is recognize that it is I who moved away from acknowledging
the connection and rejoin with the rest of God—with the rest of
myself—with you and all the rest of the universe.

I sometimes imagine that I have a fingertip of God in me, and
that you and everyone else does too. And so, we're all joined by a
great body of God. We need only remember that to feel part of the
whole again, and have knowledge and love, wisdom and beauty, healing and compassion flowing through us and between us all again.
The light and love that we feel once we have reconnected is beyond
our wildest human imaginings. The reality of our reunion with the
divine is so complete and overwhelming in its beauty, that the eu-
phoric outpouring needs to be experienced to be believed. The lack
of separateness, the flowing in, the merging with the Divine, the feel-

ing of dissolving, the timelessness, the infinity. Words can only touch on what Ramakrishna, the yogi and religious reformer, has called "a steady flow of undiluted bliss."

Living in Love with God

Throughout the ages, many have alluded to a feeling of romance, of falling in love with God.

When I was 16 and searching for my spirituality, which I appeared to have lost for a while, I changed religion. I spent every minute I could in church as my soul fell in love with the God I seemed to be able to find only there. For a brief while I toyed with the idea of spending my life in religious service since when I wasn't in church I had a deep, painful longing in my heart.

When I eventually fell in love, I came to recognize as similar that longing I felt when separated from the person I was in love with. That feeling of being in love with God has sustained me throughout my life, whatever has happened to me. And though at times I've been focused elsewhere and for awhile I may have neglected my beloved God, the relationship has always been there, holding me and being the place to which I return when I've experimented, researched, got lost in other things for awhile. As in all good relationships, I have had the freedom to look at other things, but always I have known where I truly belong. I return there when I'm ready and am welcomed in the warmest of embraces and with the richest of love.

The intensity of the union I feel varies from time to time, though the trend is always to a more profound union, to a greater euphoria in the return, to a more wondrous ease.

In 1999, I was teaching in Berlin at an open evening of spiritual dialogue that went on for several hours—much longer than we'd anticipated. Very late, I finally settled down to sleep in my hotel room.

But sleep was not on the agenda. It was one of those nights that I've known from time to time since early childhood, each of which I remember with reverence and joy.

I was held between sleep and wakefulness, fully aware with perfect clarity while angels filled the room. My body was light and I had a sense of floating above the bed while I was aware of not needing to breathe and of my whole being becoming limitless and universal. A feeling of weightlessness separated me from any sense of being real physically, yet everything was more real than anything else thus far in my life. There was absolute peace, where I had infinite knowledge and a sense of union with God and all of creation while I was held securely in a constant stream of love.

I awoke the next morning after a very brief sleep with renewed strength, purpose and direction, feeling that I'd spent a lifetime in a celestial spa! I also felt some embarrassment at ever having tried to articulate in human terms something so indescribable, limitless, infinite and powerful, but so sweet and gentle as my soul flowed out to meet it.

I knew that morning that I was once again changed forever. I had crossed a threshold—the latest and greatest in a series of encounters with God over more than 50 years. God had picked me up and powerfully changed me.

Living in love with God eventually becomes the only way to be. The spiritual journey becomes the only one to tread—transformative and peaceful—though as human beings we're likely to fall off the path now and then and find ourselves sidetracked by life events that distract us. The psyche matures as the spiritual journey unfolds and our potential is constantly revealed to be greater than we could have imagined. And with a child's eyes we see everything that comes into our path as a chance for learning and for more profound understanding of the nature of divinity, and every transaction as an opportunity to share our spirituality and love.

What's so awe-inspiring is the realization that while we've been searching for God, God has been searching for us also. It's rather like the ceiling of the Sistine Chapel—we only need to hold out our hand and there close by is the hand of God ready to touch our own. Having reconnected, the world seems a different place where there's no separation and we feel that unity consciousness we talked about earlier as a constant state. Recognizing the loving power of the spirit within us brings with it an awesome responsibility. We're committed to sharing love and peace, exemplifying the radiance of living spiritually joyous lives and helping others, so that others can learn to touch that same peace.

But none of us, unless we've already achieved sainthood, can live in peace all the time. And, as the writer Phyllis McGinley said, "The wonderful thing about saints is that they were human. They lost their tempers, scolded God, were egotistical or testy or impatient in their turns, made mistakes and regretted them. Still they went on doggedly blundering towards heaven." All you can do is try to think, pause and act rather than reacting with negative emotion, to send love where previously you may have sent anger, peace where you may have sent fear, and to deal self-assertively with what happens in your life so that petty resentments have less chance to develop. The onus is upon us to keep channels of communication open to those around us and to God.

The Love of God—a Two-Way Street

I have a somewhat irreverent relationship with God that I hope is rather refreshing to her. First of all I think God should be allowed to have some fun like the rest of us, and I think we should be able to ask questions, be angry at what happens and vent our feelings when things appear to go wrong. And we don't have to be pious all the time. What kind of a relationship would that be? I also know that God wants to keep contact with me too and desires love and communication with me. It really is a two-way street, as all loving relationships are.

How sad for us and for God that we've often been scattered, separated from each other by manmade etiquette! The "fire and brimstone" approach has done nothing but give God bad press! Who gave humankind the authority to act as an intermediary when God was happy for us to just chat with him individually? Being patronized in this way has pushed us to stand up and claim our right to be powerful, Divine beings unwilling to be disempowered by any human who attempts to decree otherwise.

I'm sure that any "hell" we've made doesn't have the approval of God. So please get up off your knees and claim your connection. No matter what we have done, how horrendous an act may appear, we still only have to reopen the door that we may have closed long ago and God's there waiting for us with the same loving welcome as always.

The more we learn to maintain our connection, the stronger, more loving and peaceful we feel in our everyday lives. The more loving and peaceful we feel, the more secure we feel and the less we need defense from the outer world and the more healed and healing we can become. But we keep coming back to the fact that we're human, aren't perfect yet and can't completely dissociate ourselves from the pain and mess of the world. But, as we discussed in the previous chapter, we don't have to court it or actively ingest it.

The Golden Rule

The golden rule is to do unto others as you would have them do unto you. This very simple statement contains the basis of living a good and inspired life. For unless we're sick or our thinking is perverse, we generally want others to be kind and gentle, honest and

Giving to receive

Imagine a huge river, constantly flowing, the water never ceasing, moving onward and constantly replaced. Spiritual love is like that. We can give it away forever and it's constantly replaced. The river never runs dry and it's important never to dam the flow, for the fresh supply brings new gifts ceaselessly. If ever we refuse to give, the flow slows and eventually stagnation results. Though the love of God will always be there, we'll cease to feel the sparkling bubbling joy if we don't let our river flow.

trustworthy, to understand us, be patient, kind and charitable towards us, to love us and let us be in peace. These gifts of the spirit we should give to others, and ultimately make manifest in our total being.

A good way to start is to check as often as you can remember to see where you're really coming from in what you say and do, being honest with yourself about your motives. If your motives are unclear, then check with your integrity. If we're in line with our true purpose, there's usually a crystal clarity about where we are, whereas any compromise to our integrity will feel dull and uncomfortable, heavy and uneasy. We need to adjust things slightly (or sometimes radically) to the point where we feel comfortable again, then proceed.

Human Love Versus Divine Love

Recapping on love in the human sense, we recall that though we may be sidetracked by physical beauty or sexual attraction, in the end we love for characteristics that are enduring and our mutual love becomes a spiritual experience. From the heart chakra and its group consciousness, we ascend to the crown with its universal consciousness and universal love. This divine love lifts us to a level beyond which ego can be involved. Attempts to describe its magnificence in human language

are doomed to failure. Only envisioning an infinite, boundless manifestation of the love we already feel begins to give us some idea of
the encompassing, endless radiance of divine love. Desire and discrimination no longer exist; simply awareness and joy and light that shines
into our souls. We are aware that God is within us and that therefore
we, with every other part of the universe, *are* God. Simultaneously
we're set in our place in the world and yet freed in the cosmos—that
undifferentiated, ordered, yet ever-changing universal soup in which
we exist—aware that, whether saint or "criminal," we're all guides
and healers. No one is more enlightened, no one more deserving or
saintly. We're all just at different points demonstrating different aspects of love to each other, everyone committed to the ultimate universal divinity of us all.

Transformation and Transcendence— Finding Heaven

One of the first rules we learn in physics at school is that matter can
neither be created nor destroyed, and that law remains true. In some
form, we've been here forever and will continue to be forever—though
our physical being is transformed. And while remaining in our human
state we can learn by meditation to enter a new dimension where
we're no longer fettered by a physical body but free to explore in a
timeless space unlimited universal consciousness. Here we can transcend any restrictions, physical or otherwise, we've created. Here we
can travel into the past, the future, observe the world from a totally
different perspective and learn new truth. Everything and everyone
you can now see in their true splendor as manifestations of love.

Here nothing is beyond you. Nothing is without value. Everything becomes an expression of love, part of a symphony, concordant
and harmonious. There's absolute clarity and you know that you'll
never be the same again, because you've entered the place of God and

are transformed. Perhaps for the first time, you can see who you are and your unlimited potential, which you may not even have suspected. This is beyond ego and pride. You're in a different dimension. One shared by divas and angels, masters and prophets. It is the realm of God.

Meditation

Take yourself to your safe place and get comfortable. As you've done so many times now, focus on your breathing and become peaceful and calm, allowing anything negative simply to flow out through the soles of your feet and your root chakra. Allow your heart to open and fill with a sweet anticipation. Let love flow throughout your body, swirling in your aura and filling the space around you. Know that there is light around you protecting you. Ask that angelic presences come to witness your ascent. Feel their love.

Allow yourself time just to be in the love. When you're ready, take your focus up now through all your chakras and out through the top of your head, through your crown chakra, gently rise now. Let yourself go: you will be safe and held in love.

Rise up and up.

Gently now, feel yourself float up to the doorway to the divine realms. You may feel almost as though you gently bump against it and with a loving breath, let it open and enter. Expand and explore. Feel the wonder and beauty of the connection with the Divine. You are experiencing your God-self rejoined to the great body of universal consciousness that is God. You may feel something reach down to meet you and hold you. Know that it will hold you loving-ly and securely and never let go . . . only you can sever the connection.

Ask anything you want to ask now. Listen for any message. Trust whatever loving communication you become aware of.

Stay as long as you wish. Know that you can return here whenever you wish and that your access will become easier and the connection stronger the more often you make it. Enjoy.

But finally you must return, for this earthly place is, for the moment, where you belong though you may transcend whenever you wish. So give thanks now and start your descent. Take your time.

Gently move back now to your crown chakra and enter again. Feel yourself becoming grounded. Be sure that you are completely back in your body. Take your time. When you are completely there, imagine a white flower above the top of your head—a thousand-petalled lotus, and with a thought, allow its petals to close now. Let your focus drop to your brow, and let the deep blue flower you will find there close also. Let your focus drop to your throat and let the blue flower there close into a bud. Let your focus drop to your heart and let the green flower you'll find there close also.

At your solar plexus you will see a bright yellow flower. Let its petals close into a tight bud and let your focus fall to your sacral chakra where, with a breath, the orange flower you'll find there will close also. Your root chakra remains open to keep you forever grounded.

Beside you, you'll find a dark blue cloak. Put it around you now and pull up the hood. Know that the light that protects you is forever with you.

Start to be aware of your breathing. Feel your fingers and toes and move them gently. Come back to a place behind your eyes and when you're ready, gently open them. Stretch a little and have a glass of water. When you're ready, record whatever you wish in your journal.

Know that you are greatly loved. That every relationship in your life can be changed irrevocably by the love in your heart. And in the words of an ancient Irish blessing:

May the road rise up to meet you,
may the wind be always at your back,
may the sun shine warm upon your face,
and the rain fall soft upon your fields,
and until we meet again
may God hold you in the palm of his hand.

Appendices

Incest

♨

*S*adly, incest is much more common than anyone would like to believe, and many cases never come to the attention of anyone outside the family. Many sufferers never even tell other family members despite the fact that the abuse may go on for several years.

Whether it is a single incident, or something repeated throughout the whole of childhood and beyond, incest is traumatic and spiritually damaging for all involved. Though on rare occasions there may appear to be a loving element, in the vast majority of cases there is threat, manipulation and often frank violence. Incest may seem to begin in "play" but it develops into a humiliating and frightening situation from which there appears to be no escape.

Though most commonly incest is between father and daughter or stepfather to stepdaughter, it can also be between mother and son, father and son or mother and daughter. Sibling incest sometimes develops as two siblings of close age get involved in sexual play, though sometimes a brother uses his much younger sister as a first sexual partner. At times members of the extended family are involved, such as uncles and grandfathers, and occasionally it becomes almost a family tradition with several members of the family performing sexual acts with the children. In some families several daughters will be involved one after the other, leading to considerable guilt among them—the older ones regretting not protecting the younger ones by telling someone, or being relieved when their father moves on to a younger child, perhaps when the possibility of pregnancy arises. The relationship between the siblings is always damaged as the element of protection of each other is lost and is replaced by a sense of betrayal.

In the family where there is incest all relationships are damaged. Children feel betrayed by the parent who commits the crime, but also by the other parent who does nothing to protect them—whether out of ignorance or out of cowardice or even relief that the sexual pressure is at least off them.

We looked at acting-out behavior in Chapter 5, where children will show us that something is wrong even though they may not be able to communicate their distress verbally. Incest is most commonly dealt with in this way. In the short term, changes in behavior such as a child becoming nervous, sullen, withdrawn, disruptive or angry and being afraid to be left alone may indicate that something is wrong. Changes in performance at school, bed-wetting, aggressive play or play of a sexual nature need to be gently explored.

Almost always there are long-term consequences. Children are taught to deny their feelings and sometimes they become unable to feel at all, becoming locked and frozen in a sea of guilt, shame and numbness. They learn not to talk about what is hurting them, to pretend, and are often told that what is happening is their fault (which it *never* is), so the development of the personality is distorted.

In adulthood, personality disorders are common among incest survivors, with drinking, drug taking and violence becoming part of their lives. They are often self-destructive, with self-harm and suicide attempts. They also enter into repeated destructive relationships where they may be the victims of violence—physical, emotional or spiritual.

Sometimes they themselves become the aggressor in such relationships, and victims of abuse often become abusers themselves, though the form may vary. Victims of incest may have difficulty with their control of anger and may find themselves physically abusing their partners or even their own children. There are almost always sexual problems including seductive and promiscuous behavior and sometimes prostitution or repression of sexual desire, with frigidity. They are often jealous and suspicious. Unplanned and unwanted pregnancies are common, often not in the context of a committed relationship. Many women who have suffered sexual abuse develop eating disorders.

Breaking the silence about incest is a painful process and many women (and men) never do so. Some women in their late sixties or even seventies have finally talked to me about what went on in their homes, sharing the shame they have been carrying for decades. Sometimes one sister will have the courage to talk about her problem to find that her sisters have also suffered similarly though each thought they were protecting the others and carrying the burden alone. The secret may be revealed only when a daughter refuses to allow her child to be alone with his grandfather lest the abuse be continued down the generations.

There are always issues of grief and abandonment, the pain of not having been protected by the parents whose job it was to do so, though often the abused child fiercely protects the non-abusing parent rather than accept that they might have been betrayed by both.

If there has been incest in your family, whether or not you were involved, it would be wise for you to find some professional help. Sometimes there is complete repression of memory (it's as though it never happened) but when the repression starts to lift, as it may when there is a crisis in your life or some event such as having a baby, or someone dying, or you read a newspaper article about abuse, flashbacks—snatches of memory about what happened to you—

might start to occur. The fact that you have "forgotten" the abuse for decades doesn't mean it didn't happen. Do get some good professional help. Ongoing support is available and is essential for many who are trying to come to terms with this dreadful part of their past that is getting in the way of them having a pleasant life. The fact that it ruined your early life doesn't mean that it has to go on spoiling the rest of your life.

There are several good books which would also help you:

Ellen Bass and Laura Davis, *The Courage to Heal*, Cedar, 1988.

Louise M. Wisechild, *The Obsidian Mirror*, Seal Press, 1988.

Eliana Gil, *The Treatment of Adult Survivors of Childhood Abuse*, Launch Press, 1990.

And particularly for men:

Mike Lew, *Victims No Longer*, HarperCollins, 1990.

Past Lives

I have been here before,
But when or how I cannot tell:
I know the grass beyond the door,
The sweet keen smell,
The sighing sound, the lights around the shore.
You have been mine before—
How long ago I may not know:
But just when at that swallow's soar
Your neck turned so,
Some veil did fall—I knew it all of yore.
Has this been thus before?
And shall not thus time's eddying flight
Still with our lives our love restore
In death's despite,
And the day and night yield one delight once more?

—Dante Gabriel Rossetti, "Sudden Light"

Shakespeare, Kipling, Wordsworth, Benjamin Franklin and General Patton are but a few of those who have talked openly about their knowledge of past-life connections and the continuity of life.

Even Jesus told the apostles that John the Baptist was a reincarnation of earlier prophets.

There is considerable evidence from many sources, both anecdotal and scientific, that we have lived before. Since 1967, the Department of Psychiatric Medicine of the University of Virginia has carried out investigations of paranormal phenomena and several books have been published on their work. Some titles of these and other books on the subject will be found at the end of this appendix. The University of Edinburgh, the University of Hertfordshire, Princeton University and the University of Amsterdam are studying similar phenomena.

Having worked with many people who have come to terms with events in this lifetime by searching the past, I have no doubt whatsoever that we have lived many lifetimes and will probably live many more. I have evidence in my own life of many places where I have lived before and of some of those people with whom I have lived. Many are with me again in this lifetime, and will be again.

Over many years, children from various parts of the world have reported memories of past lives, often being able to describe clearly where they lived before, who they were, what happened in their lives and how they died. Often such memories cease by the age of about five or six, though sometimes the children carry with them phobias, skills or physical markings that cannot be explained by events of this lifetime but link closely with what they have reported. Many of these children have been investigated and found to have knowledge that they could not possibly have gained in their current life. Though many adults are unaware of any such memory, they may find themselves with unexplained symptoms which are difficult to treat and remove but that can be traced back to another time.

Sometimes with advancing age and an interest in spiritual matters, there is emerging memory of who we were. Interests, passions and talents may call us. We may feel we have a special affinity with a place or race, feel at home with them and sense a deep connection. We might find ourselves collecting artifacts from a particular place or time and feel a strange longing in our hearts when touching them or even reading about them. We may visit a new place and feel that we've been there before, not simply as a momentary déjà vu, but as a deep knowing that moves us. In meeting new people, particularly those with whom we fall in love or become good friends, there may be a sense of having known them before. Perhaps someone in your original family with whom you have either an extremely close connection or an acrimonious one may have lived with you before. Occasionally we may have an unexplained aversion to someone who has done us no harm, but with whom we feel anxious and ill at ease, even afraid. There is a possibility that we have been in some way associated in a not very pleasant transaction in the past. Similarly, we may find ourselves with unexplained discomfort on visiting a particular place or entering a building, and it may be that we have been there before too in a less-than-happy time.

Karma is the process by which we balance our books as it were; a cycle of cause and effect that eventually brings us to a state of balance. Karma is continuous through all lifetimes and therefore we may bring with us unfinished business that we need to deal with. We have all done good things and bad in our past. We have lived through ages where deeds were acceptable that would fill us with horror today. If you are repaying some karma now, then rather than be sad about it, why not rejoice that you're making good and will never have to do so again? We repay our debts, cancel out our bad deeds by doing something better and worthwhile. We can all start from this moment to live more loving, graceful lives and cancel out whatever we may have done in the past.

Sometimes the way we live out our karma can be symbolic. For example we could choose in this life to work lovingly with deprived children to make restitution for the fact that we abandoned a child or did harm to a child in an earlier life. Sometimes we come with a direct carryover from a previous life where perhaps we died with great anger or bitterness and we come back with a similar problem so that we can learn to do it again and let go of the pain. Occasionally we choose situations that are difficult to comprehend in order to cancel out much karma in a short period of time and release ourselves to come again in peace. We often return to meet with the same souls again and again in different guises so that we can continue to learn the lessons we set ourselves; and sometimes we incarnate with souls we have never lived with.

Our soul chooses a particular set of invariables at birth (see Chapter 5) that will allow us to bring our obligations to this incarnation, to give us a head start and be in a position where we're able to fulfill them. Our parents give us characteristics that will help us with the process. This is what science calls heredity or genetic predisposition. In fact, our parents are chosen wisely by us to help us set the scene and launch us into our chosen life.

Our temperaments vary considerably, and while some live on the surface and are uninterested in why things are as they are, others have restless, passionate, curious minds constantly searching for answers. If you were one of the former, you wouldn't be reading this book.

SOUL MATES

We talked a little of soul mates in Chapter 8. There are several kinds of soul mates—including soul twins, companion soul mates and the karmic soul mates. Soul mates need not necessarily be heterosexual, nor even sexual partners at all. Sometimes we find a soul mate in a dear, anciently beloved friend. Though some may think in terms of one eternal soul with one eternal mate for that soul, that's not necessarily how it is—though it may be for some.

There is evidence that we may live in parallel universes, living out parts of ourselves simultaneously in different geographical locations with different soul mates in each one. And in a single lifetime we may meet again more than one soul mate or may never meet one—though that doesn't mean that we don't have deeply loving and satisfying relationships.

FURTHER READING

There are many texts that will intrigue and excite you and you may also want to come along to a past-life workshop or find a reputable therapist to undertake some past-life work with you. You may like to refer to the useful information on page 303, and may find some of the following books interesting.

Gina Germinara, *Many Mansions*, Signet, 1991.
Elisabeth Haich, *Initiation*, Seed Center, 1974 (difficult to obtain, but worth looking for).
Dr. Ian Stevenson, *Children Who Remember Previous Lives*, McFarland & Company, 2000.
Dr. Brian L. Weiss, *Many Lives, Many Masters*, Simon & Schuster, 1988.
Dr. Brian L. Weiss, *Through Time into Healing*, Simon & Schuster, 1992.

Depression Checklist

✤

Depression can be insidious or hit us like a bolt out of the blue. However, it's very treatable and even though you may feel that there's nothing that can be done, there usually is. But the first move needs to be yours in being willing to go along to your doctor and ask for help. For some kinds of depression you may need medication; for some, therapy. You can always help yourself by having nurturing treatments like massage, aromatherapy, homeopathy, reflexology, etc. But if your brain chemistry is upset and you need an orthodox antidepressant, then accept it because it will enable you to deal with the other things in life that you need to change. (See *Total Wellbeing*, by Dr. Hilary Jones and Dr. Brenda Davies).

You'd be wise to ask for help if you persistently:
- feel despair
- cry a lot
- feel anxious much of the time
- worry about things
- feel low in energy
- have little interest in family, household, work, etc.

- have difficulty having fun
- find it hard to laugh
- wish you wouldn't wake up tomorrow
- wish you were dead
- have little interest in food or eat to comfort yourself
- have lost weight without trying
- have little interest in sex
- feel irritable, angry a lot of the time
- have little impulse control
- have difficulty in concentrating
- feel guilty or ashamed
- feel stuck in the past and can't move on
- have thoughts of wanting to harm or kill yourself
- avoid eye contact because it feels painful to look people in the eye
- sit staring into space with little going on in your mind
- feel pestered by thoughts that go round and round in your mind
- wake earlier than usual
- can't get to sleep at night
- feel dreadful in the morning even though by evening you don't feel so bad
- feel worse in the evening even though the morning wasn't too bad
- feel hopeless, as though there's nothing to live for
- feel that you'll never be okay again
- feel as though you've lost your self-confidence and self-esteem
- have lost interest in your appearance
- are drinking too much

Do have a professional assessment and think of having someone to talk with while you're working on yourself. If therapy isn't possible for you, how about setting up your own study group to work through *Unlocking the Heart Chakra*. You could support each other and do the meditations together.

Whatever you do, take care of yourself.

Bibliography

Dr. Robert Ackerman, *Silent Sons*, Thorsons, 1994.

Carolyn Ainscough and Kay Toon, *Breaking Free*, Sheldon Press, 1993.

The Confessions of St. Augustine, translated by the Most Reverend Fulton J. Sheen, DD, Random House, 1949.

Ellen Bass and Laura Davis, *Courage to Heal*, Cedar, 1988.

M'haletta and Carmella B'Hahn, *Benjaya's Gifts*, Hazelwood Press, 1996.

Dietrich Bonhoeffer, *Letters and Papers from Prison*, SCM Press, 1953.

J. Allen Boone, *Kinship with All Life*, Harper & Row, 1954.

Barbara Brennan, *Hands of Light*, Bantam, 1987.

Betty Burzon Ph.D., *Permanent Partners*, Plume, 1988.

Leo Buscaglia, *Love*, Fawcett Crest, 1972.

Dwight L. Carlson, M.D., *Overcoming Hurts and Anger*, Harvest House, 1981.

Paul M. Conner, O.P., *Celibate Love*, Our Sunday Visitor, Inc., 1978.

Dr. Brenda Davies, *The 7 Healing Chakras*, Ulysses Press, 2000.

Bill Defoore, *Anger: Deal With It, Heal With It, Stop It From Killing You*, Deerfield Beach, 1991.

Gentry W. Doyle, *Anger Free—Ten Basic Steps to Managing Your Anger*, W. Morrison & Co., 1999.

The Foundation for Inner Peace, *A Course in Miracles*, Arkana Press, 1996.

Victor Emil Frankl, *Recollections—An Autobiography*, Insight Books Inc., 1997.

Kahlil Gibran, *The Prophet*, Heinemann, 1926.

Eliana Gil, *The Treatment of Adult Survivors of Childhood Abuse*, Launch Press, 1990.

Jean Houston, *In Search of the Beloved*, Jeremy P. Tarcher, 1987.

Gerald Jampolsky, *Love Is Letting Go of Fear*, Celestial Arts, 1982.

Dr. Hilary Jones and Dr. Brenda Davies, *Total Wellbeing—The Whole Treatment for the Whole You*, Hodder & Stoughton, 1999.

Sam Keene, *To Love and Be Loved*, Bantam, 1997.

R.D. Laing, *The Politics of Experience*, Pantheon, 1967.

John Lee, *At My Father's Wedding*, Bantam, 1991.

John Lee, *The Flying Boy*, Health Communication, 1987.

Mike Lew, *Victims No Longer*, HarperCollins, 1990.

Roger McGough, *Defying Gravity*, Penguin, 1992.

Eric Marcus, *Is It a Choice?*, HarperCollins, 1999.

Nikhilnanda, *Ramakrishna: Prophet of New India*, Harper & Row, 1948.

Dorothy Law Nolte and Rachel Harris, *Children Learn What They Live: Parenting to Inspire Values*, Workman Publishing Company, 1998.

John O'Donohue, *Anam Cara*, Bantam Press, 1997.

James Redfield, *The Secret of Shambhala*, Warner, 1999.

Antoine de Saint-Exupéry, *The Little Prince*, Heinemann, 1945 edn.

Antoine de Saint-Exupéry, *Wind, Sand and Stars*, Harcourt Brace, 1967 edn.

Brenda Schaeffer, *Is It Love Or Is It Addiction?* Hazelden, 1987.

Victoria Secunda, *Women and Their Fathers*, Delacorte Press, 1992.

Jess Stearn, *Soul Mates*, Bantam, 1984.

Neale Donald Walsch, *Conversations with God, Volumes 1, 2 and 3*, Hodder & Stoughton, 1997.

James Q. Wilson, *The Moral Sense*, The Free Press, 1993.

Louise M. Wisechild, *The Obsidian Mirror*, Seal Press, 1988.

Useful Addresses

To order affirmation cards, massage oils, meditation tapes, CDs and other holistic products:

By mail:

    The Brenda Davies Collection

    P.O. Box 803, Weimar, Texas 78962

By internet:

    products@brendadavies-collection.com

    For details of workshops and seminars or

    to book Dr. Brenda Davies to speak at conferences etc.

By mail:

    Brenda Davies Seminars, P.O. Box 803, Weimar, Texas 78962

By internet:

    workshops@brendadavies-collection.com

Other Ulysses Press Mind/Body Titles

BEAUTY SECRETS OF INDIA: FROM AYURVEDIC TECHNIQUES
TO EXOTIC ADORNMENTS
Monisha Bharadwaj, $17.95

The author, born and raised in Bombay, captures this romantic realm with a personal, easy-going style that includes family recipes and girlfriend tips.

CHAKRA POWER BEADS: TAPPING THE POWER OF HEALING STONES
TO UNLOCK YOUR INNER POTENTIAL
Brenda Davies, $9.95

Explains how to improve health, spirit and fortune by fully harnessing the *power* of beads.

GIVE YOUR FACE A LIFT: NATURAL WAYS TO LOOK AND FEEL GOOD
Penny Stanway, $17.95

This full-color guide to natural face care tells how to give oneself a "natural facelift" using oils, creams, masks and homemade products that nourish and beautify the skin.

HEALING REIKI: REUNITE MIND, BODY AND SPIRIT WITH HEALING ENERGY
Eleanor McKenzie, $16.95

Examines the meaning, attitudes and history of Reiki while providing practical tips for receiving and giving this universal life energy.

HERBS THAT WORK: THE SCIENTIFIC EVIDENCE OF THEIR HEALING POWERS
David Armstrong, $12.95

Unlike herb books relying on folklore or vague anecdotes, *Herbs that Work* is the first consumer guide to rate herbal remedies based on documented, state-of-the-art scientific research.

HOW MEDITATION HEALS: A PRACTICAL GUIDE TO IMPROVING
YOUR HEALTH AND WELL-BEING
Eric Harrison, $12.95

Combines Eastern wisdom with medical and scientific evidence to explain how and why meditation improves the functioning of all systems of the body.

HOW TO MEDITATE: AN ILLUSTRATED GUIDE TO CALMING THE MIND AND
RELAXING THE BODY
Paul Roland, $16.95

Offers a friendly, illustrated approach to calming the mind and raising consciousness through various techniques, including basic meditation, visualization, body scanning for tension, affirmations and mantras.

THE JOSEPH H. PILATES METHOD AT HOME:
A BALANCE, SHAPE, STRENGTH & FITNESS PROGRAM
Eleanor McKenzie, $16.95

This handbook describes and details Pilates, a mental and physical program that combines elements of yoga and classical dance.

KNOW YOUR BODY: THE ATLAS OF ANATOMY
2nd edition, Introduction by Emmet B. Keeffe, M.D., $14.95

Provides a comprehensive, full-color guide to the human body.

MAGNET THERAPY ILLUSTRATED: NATURAL HEALING
AND PAIN RELIEF USING MAGNETS
Peter Rose, $11.95

Mixes need-to-know facts with how-to techniques to let readers immediately tap the healing power of magnets.

SENSES WIDE OPEN: THE ART AND PRACTICE OF LIVING IN YOUR BODY
Johanna Putnoi, $14.95

Through simple, accessible exercises, this book shows how to be at ease with yourself and experience genuine pleasure in your physical connection to others and the world.

THE 7 HEALING CHAKRAS: UNLOCKING YOUR BODY'S ENERGY CENTERS
Brenda Davies, $14.95

Explores the essence of chakras, vortices of energy that connect the physical body with the spiritual.

SIMPLY RELAX: AN ILLUSTRATED GUIDE TO SLOWING DOWN
AND ENJOYING LIFE
Dr. Sarah Brewer, $15.95

In a beautifully illustrated format, this book clearly presents physical and mental disciplines that show readers how to relax.

WEEKEND HOME SPA: FOUR CREATIVE ESCAPES—CLEANSING, ENERGIZING,
RELAXING AND PAMPERING
Linda Bird, $16.95

Shows how to create that spa experience in your own home with step-by-step mini workouts, stretching routines, meditations and visualizations, as well as more challenging exercises to boost mental potential.

To order these books call 800-377-2542 or 510-601-8301, fax 510-601-8307, e-mail ulysses@ulyssespress.com, or write to Ulysses Press, P.O. Box 3440, Berkeley, CA 94703. All retail orders are shipped free of charge. California residents must include sales tax. Allow two to three weeks for delivery.